HUMAN DEVELOPMENT, RELATIONSHIPS, AND SEXUAL HEALTH

ESSENTIAL
Health Skills for Middle School

FOURTH EDITION

Catherine A. Sanderson, PhD
Professor of Psychology
Amherst College
Amherst, Massachusetts

Mark Zelman, PhD
Professor of Biology
Aurora University
Aurora, Illinois

PEDAGOGY DEVELOPERS

Lindsay R. Armbruster
Health Education Teacher
Burnt Hills, New York

Mary McCarley
National Health Education Content Specialist
National Board Certified Teacher in Health Education
Charlotte, North Carolina

Publisher
The Goodheart-Willcox Company, Inc.
Tinley Park, IL
www.g-w.com

Copyright © 2025
by
The Goodheart-Willcox Company, Inc.

Previous editions copyright 2019, 2021, 2023

All rights reserved. No part of this work may be reproduced, stored, or transmitted in any form or by any electronic or mechanical means, including information storage and retrieval systems, except as permitted by U.S. copyright law, without the prior written permission of The Goodheart-Willcox Company, Inc.

ISBN 979-8-88817-929-1

2 3 4 5 6 7 8 9 – 25 – 28 27 26 25 24

The Goodheart-Willcox Company, Inc. Brand Disclaimer: Brand names, company names, and illustrations for products and services included in this text are provided for educational purposes only and do not represent or imply endorsement or recommendation by the author or the publisher.

The Goodheart-Willcox Company, Inc. CDC Disclaimer: The use of materials from the CDC (Centers for Disease Control and Prevention) used in Goodheart-Willcox textbooks and supplements does not imply endorsement or recommendation by the CDC, ATSDR (Agency for Toxic Substances and Disease Registry), HHS (Department of Health and Human Services), or the United States Government for the content, products, or services contained in Goodheart-Willcox print or digital publications. Materials from the CDC are also available at http://www.cdc.gov free of charge.

The Goodheart-Willcox Company, Inc. Safety Notice: The reader is expressly advised to carefully read, understand, and apply all safety precautions and warnings described in this book or that might also be indicated in undertaking the activities and exercises described herein to minimize risk of personal injury or injury to others. Common sense and good judgment should also be exercised and applied to help avoid all potential hazards. The reader should always refer to the appropriate manufacturer's technical information, directions, and recommendations; then proceed with care to follow specific equipment operating instructions. The reader should understand these notices and cautions are not exhaustive.

The publisher makes no warranty or representation whatsoever, either expressed or implied, including but not limited to equipment, procedures, and applications described or referred to herein, their quality, performance, merchantability, or fitness for a particular purpose. The publisher assumes no responsibility for any changes, errors, or omissions in this book. The publisher specifically disclaims any liability whatsoever, including any direct, indirect, incidental, consequential, special, or exemplary damages resulting, in whole or in part, from the reader's use or reliance upon the information, instructions, procedures, warnings, cautions, applications, or other matter contained in this book. The publisher assumes no responsibility for the activities of the reader.

The Goodheart-Willcox Company, Inc. Internet Disclaimer: The Internet resources and listings in this Goodheart-Willcox Publisher product are provided solely as a convenience to you. These resources and listings were reviewed at the time of publication to provide you with accurate, safe, and appropriate information. Goodheart-Willcox Publisher has no control over the referenced websites and, due to the dynamic nature of the Internet, is not responsible or liable for the content, products, or performance of links to other websites or resources. Goodheart-Willcox Publisher makes no representation, either expressed or implied, regarding the content of these websites, and such references do not constitute an endorsement or recommendation of the information or content presented. It is your responsibility to take all protective measures to guard against inappropriate content, viruses, or other destructive elements.

Image Credits: Front cover: SerrNovik/iStock/Getty Images Plus via Getty Images; mmg1design/iStock/Getty Images Plus via Getty Images; Wavebreakmedia/iStock/Getty Images Plus via Getty Images

About the Authors

Catherine A. Sanderson is the Poler Family Professor of Psychology at Amherst College. She received a bachelor's degree in psychology, with a specialization in Health and Development, from Stanford University, and received both master's and doctoral degrees in psychology from Princeton University. Professor Sanderson's research examines how personality and social variables influence health-related behaviors, such as safer sex and disordered eating. Her research also examines the development of persuasive messages and interventions to prevent unhealthy behavior and predictors of relationship satisfaction. This research has received grant funding from the National Science Foundation and the National Institutes of Health. Professor Sanderson has published more than 25 journal articles and book chapters; four college textbooks; high school and middle school health textbooks; and a trade book, *The Positive Shift*, which examines how mind-set influences happiness, health, and even how long people live. Her latest book, *Why We Act: Turning Bystanders into Moral Rebels*, examines why good people often stay silent or do nothing in the face of wrongdoing. In 2012, she was named one of the country's top 300 professors by the Princeton Review.

Mark Zelman is a Professor of Biology at Aurora University, Aurora, Illinois. He received a bachelor's degree in biology from Rockford College. He received a PhD in microbiology and immunology from Loyola University of Chicago and completed a postdoctoral fellowship at the University of Chicago. Dr. Zelman's research focuses on prevention and control of infectious diseases, mechanisms of antibiotic resistance, and community factors affecting public health. He teaches science education courses for high school teachers. He has published articles on microbiology, infectious disease, autoimmune disease, and biotechnology, and he has written two college texts on human diseases and infection control. Dr. Zelman works with the West Africa AIDS Foundation in Ghana and other public health projects in the US and abroad. He is an officer of the Illinois State Academy of Sciences and Editor-in-Chief of the Academy's scientific journal, *Transactions*.

Pedagogy Developers

Lindsay Armbruster experiences on a daily basis the impact that optimism, self-efficacy, and persistence can have on a class, an individual, and on students' health behaviors. As a result, her teaching focuses on strengths and possibilities and is highly influenced by the theories of skills-based health education and positive psychology. Lindsay is certified as both a K–12 Health Education teacher and K-12 Library Media Specialist in the state of New York. Lindsay has been teaching Health Education since 2004, ranging all grade levels—kindergarten through 12th grade as well as graduate school—with most of her experience occurring at the middle school level. Lindsay received her bachelor's degree in school and community health education from the State University of New York College at Brockport and her master's degree in curriculum development and instructional technology from the University at Albany. Lindsay also earned a second master's degree in Library Media at St. John Fisher University. She has won the New York State Association for Health, Physical Education, Recreation and Dance (NYSAHPERD) Health Teacher of the Year award and the Society of Health & Physical Educators (SHAPE) America Eastern District Health Teacher of the Year award. Lindsay is a frequent presenter at local, state, and regional conferences.

Mary McCarley is the National Health Education Content Specialist. She taught health education for 14 years in Charlotte Mecklenburg Schools. As a teacher, she excelled at creating an engaging, student-centered learning environment with a focus on real-world learning and skills-based health education. Mary graduated from UNC-Chapel Hill with an Exercise and Sports Science degree and East Carolina University with a Master of Arts in Education in Health Education. She is a National Board Certified Teacher in Health Education. In addition, Mary is the 2016 North Carolina High School Teacher of the Year for Health Education and the 2016 High School Southern District Teacher of the Year for the Advancement of Health Education. Mary presents at conferences and for school districts on various health education topics locally and nationally. She provides professional development and training for school districts to help teachers effectively implement a skills-based health education curriculum.

Reviewers

Advisory Board

Goodheart-Willcox Publisher would like to thank the following advisory board members who provided guidance in the development of *Essential Health Skills for Middle School: Human Development, Relationships, and Sexual Health.*

Haillie Bell
Health and Physical Education Instructor
Sherman E. Burroughs High School
Ridgecrest, California

Melanie Busch
Health and Physical Education Instructor
Homestead High School
Fort Wayne, Indiana

Cyndi Cain
Health Education Instructor
Champlin Park High School
Champlin, Minnesota

Amelia Chandler
Health Instructor
Anaheim Union High School District
Anaheim, California

Kimberly Clay
Health Instructor
Park Hill School District
Kansas City, Missouri

Kelly Dodd
Health Instructor
Park Hill School District
Kansas City, Missouri

Stephanie Eliasen
Health Instructor
Bondurant-Farrar Junior High School
Bondurant, Iowa

Kat Gratz
Health Instructor
Columbus East High School
Columbus, Indiana

Hilary Machemer
Health and Physical Education Instructor
Carmel Clay School District
Carmel, Indiana

Stephanie Neff
Health Instructor
Washington High School
Cedar Rapids, Iowa

Christina Olson
Health Education Instructor
Champlin Park High School
Champlin, Minnesota

Kyle Petty
Health Instructor
Washington Liberty
Arlington, Virginia

Caitlin Provance
Curriculum Coordinator
Lincoln Public Schools
Lincoln, Nebraska

Jamie Sebring
Wellness Instructor
Taft Middle School
Cedar Rapids, Iowa

Leah Swedberg
Health Instructor
West Fargo High School
West Fargo, North Dakota

Cynthia Terrell
Healthful Living Instructor
Wakefield High School
Raleigh, North Carolina

Sarah Van Berkum
Health Instructor
Anaheim Union High School District
Anaheim, California

Professional Reviewers

Goodheart-Willcox Publisher would like to thank the following health professionals who reviewed selected lessons and contributed valuable input into the development of *Essential Health Skills for Middle School: Human Development, Relationships, and Sexual Health*.

Lauren O'Sullivan
Genetic Counselor
Seattle Children's Hospital
Seattle, Washington

Shelly Vaziri Flais, MD, FAAP
Physician, Pediatrician
New Lenox, Illinois

Teacher Reviewers

Goodheart-Willcox Publisher would like to thank the following health education teachers who reviewed selected lessons and contributed valuable input into the development of *Essential Health Skills for Middle School: Human Development, Relationships, and Sexual Health*.

Jan Francis
Health Teacher
Douglas County School District
Parker, Colorado

Cheryll Hall
Health Education Teacher
Kernan Middle School/Duval
 County Public Schools
Jacksonville, Florida

Jessica Kinsey
Health and Wellness Teacher
Mammoth Heights Elementary
 School
Parker, Colorado

Contents

Module 8 Development, the Human Life Cycle, and Relationships........................ 1

- **Lesson 8.1** Human Development 2
  - Review and Assessment 8
- **Lesson 8.2** Changes During Puberty........................ 9
  - Review and Assessment 19
- **Lesson 8.3** Human Reproduction........................ 20
  - Review and Assessment 28
- **Lesson 8.4** Dating Relationships and Abstinence 29
  - Review and Assessment 10

Module 9 Violence 41

- **Lesson 9.1** Bullying and Cyberbullying........................ 42
  - Review and Assessment 54
- **Lesson 9.2** Unwanted Sexual Activity 55
  - Review and Assessment 65
- **Lesson 9.3** Abuse and Neglect 66
  - Review and Assessment 77
- **Lesson 9.4** Violence in the Community 78
  - Review and Assessment 86

Module 10 Pregnancy and STIs 87

- **Lesson 10.1** Teen Pregnancy and Parenthood 88
  - Review and Assessment 96
- **Lesson 10.2** Sexually Transmitted Infections (STIs)........................ 97
  - Review and Assessment 108
- **Lesson 10.3** HIV/AIDS 109
  - Review and Assessment 116

Module 11	Sexual Health	117
Lesson 11.1	What is Sexuality?	118
	Review and Assessment	129
Lesson 11.2	Sexual Feelings and Abstinence	130
	Review and Assessment	138
Lesson 11.3	Pregnancy Prevention	139
	Review and Assessment	150

Glossary 151

Index 158

Feature Contents

CASE STUDIES

Akiko Feels Left Behind 11	Aiden's "Perfect" Relationship 102
Jake Learns About Reproduction 25	Cameron and Tyree's Not-So-Magical Relationship 137
Martina's First Date 33	
Aarav and Rajesh: Boys Will Be Boys 73	Aparna Chooses Abstinence 142

BUILDING YOUR SKILLS | Community Connections

Peer Pressure Throughout the Life Span 18
The Importance of Consent 57
Testing and Treatment 106
Promoting Acceptance, Tolerance, and Unity 127

BUILDING YOUR SKILLS | Mental Health Connections

Making Decisions About Boundaries 95

BUILDING YOUR SKILLS | Digital Connections

Rumor Has It 46
The Impact of Sexting 134

Infographics

Puberty: What to Excpet 12
How to Spot Cyberbullying 49
Breaking the Myth of Gendered
    Personality Traits. 123
Benefits of Abstinence from Sexual Activity 143

To the Student

We wrote this exciting textbook for middle school health and wellness classes based on our experiences as professors of psychology (Catherine Sanderson) and biology (Mark Zelman), and as the accomplished authors of high school and college-level textbooks. Our backgrounds give us a deep well of knowledge of the most current scientific theory and research to draw from.

Perhaps the most valuable experience we had in preparing us to write this book is our roles as parents to a combined total of seven children, ages 15 through 29. After all, in writing this book, we both reflected frequently on our experiences as parents and our goal of ensuring that our own children maintain excellent physical, mental and emotional, and social health.

As a supplement to the textbook, we created *Essential Health Skills for Middle School: Human Development, Relationships, and Sexual Health*. Picking up where the textbook leaves off, this supplement covers topics from bullying and cyberbullying to pregnancy prevention. As with our textbook, we wanted this supplement to give middle school students the most current health information, presented in an engaging writing style so students would enjoy reading the book. Additionally, we included a focus on practical health skills that young people can use to develop and promote good health and wellness habits throughout their lives.

As the authors of high school and college-level textbooks, we felt confident in our research and writing abilities, but felt that the pedagogy was better left to health teachers. We would like to thank Lindsay Armbruster for developing the skills-based questions, activities, and resources that are a vital part of this course. We are delighted with the final product, and wish all readers of this book a lifetime of health.

Catherine A. Sanderson   Mark Zelman

Module 8: Development, the Human Life Cycle, and Relationships

- **Lesson 8.1** Human Development
- **Lesson 8.2** Changes During Puberty
- **Lesson 8.3** Human Reproduction
- **Lesson 8.4** Dating Relationships and Abstinence

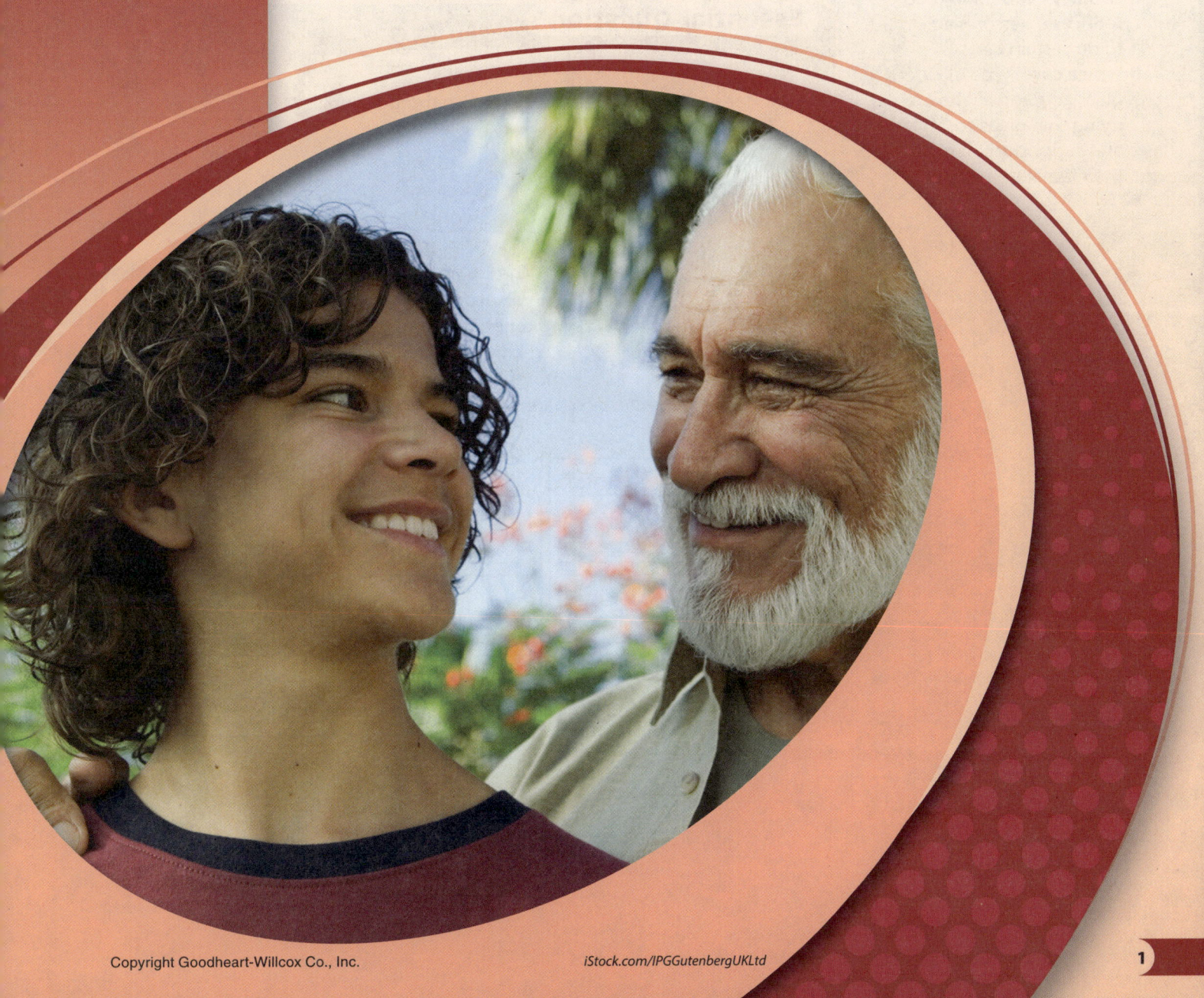

Lesson 8.1 Human Development

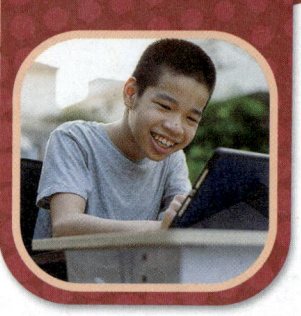

Key Terms

human life cycle sequence of developmental stages from birth through adulthood

life span number of years a person lives

life expectancy estimate of how long a person in a particular society is likely to live

disability condition that reduces a person's ability to do certain tasks

hospice care type of care given to people who are dying that gives comfort and support to them and their families

Learning Outcomes

Look for the skills icon  to practice health skills.
After studying this lesson, you will be able to

8.1–1 **Identify** the different areas of development in the human life cycle.
8.1–2 **Describe** the factors that influence development.
8.1–3 **Explain** the end of life and how people can cope with grief and loss.

Essential Question

How does a person develop and change throughout life?

Reading and Notetaking Activity

Throughout the human life cycle, a person will experience physical, intellectual, emotional, and social changes. As you read this lesson, use an organizer to take notes about the human life cycle, the various developments and changes that occur during a person's life, and the end of life.

The Human Life Cycle	Human Development	The End of Life
•	•	•
•	•	•
•	•	•

Goodheart-Willcox Publisher

Lesson image:
Ann Gaysorn/Shutterstock.com

Introduction

Destiny remembers watching her little brother grow from an infant into a young child. Destiny also recognizes the changes that she has gone through herself in childhood. She has grown several inches, learned how to be a good friend, and started to build her self-esteem.

A human life is made up of stages like a book is made up of chapters. The story of a life unfolds in the same way that chapters build on each other. In this lesson, you will learn about the chapters of life. You will also learn how each person's story and development is different.

8.1-1 The Human Life Cycle

When a baby is born, the **human life cycle** begins. This cycle is a sequence of developmental stages from birth through adulthood. With each new stage, the person begins a new phase of life. These life stages are shown in **Figure 8.1.1**.

Essential Idea

The human life cycle is made of stages, and each life cycle is unique.

Stages of the Human Life Cycle

Stage	Development	Stage	Development
Early childhood (Infancy, from birth to one year. Toddler, from one to three. Preschool, from three to five.) *Marlon Lopez MMG1 Design/Shutterstock.com*	Rapid physical growth; forming emotional connections and empathy; learning to walk, run, and kick a ball; feeding themselves; and learning to talk	**Middle childhood** (Five to 12 years of age) *Marlon Lopez MMG1 Design/Shutterstock.com*	Continued physical growth, either slow and steady or in spurts; learning to problem-solve and think logically; forming friendships and other relationships; and developing self-esteem and confidence
Adolescence (12 to 19 years of age) *santypan/Shutterstock.com*	Maturing of reproductive systems (puberty); beginning of menstruation; increasing independence; learning to think through complex problems and think more abstractly; becoming concerned about the acceptance of peers	**Adulthood** (Twenty years of age and older) *Click Images/Shutterstock.com*	Reaching end of physical growth and start of physical decline; becoming better at managing emotions and stress; experiencing new emotional relationships such as in marriages and those with children

Figure 8.1.1 Looking at your baby pictures and school photos together will show how much you have changed already in your life cycle.

Each person's life cycle is unique. The length of each stage can differ slightly for each person. People also have different life spans. A **life span** is the number of years a person lives. A person's life span may be affected by the following factors:

- genetic makeup
- environment
- lifestyle, including making healthy choices or taking part in risky behaviors
- certain diseases
- regular healthcare

Life expectancy is an estimate of how long a person in a society is likely to live. Life expectancy differs from one country to another. It can also differ for groups in the same country, based on a variety of factors (**Figure 8.1.2**). In the United States, the life expectancy is 73.2 years for males and 79.1 years for females. The overall health of a society affects life expectancy. For example, the COVID-19 pandemic and drug overdoses have recently reduced life expectancy in the United States.

Figure 8.1.2 Certain factors can change a person's life expectancy.

Does education increase or decrease life expectancy?

What Affects Life Expectancy?

Increases Life Expectancy
Education, income, clean environment, healthcare

Decreases Life Expectancy
Pollution, violence, poverty, disease

Goodheart-Willcox Publisher

8.1–1 Reading Checkpoint

1. List the stages of the human life cycle. What stage of life are you in?
2. A person's life expectancy is affected by several factors. What factors positively and negatively influence life expectancy?

Essential Idea

Physical, intellectual, emotional, and social development are often related and affect each other. Differences in development are common.

8.1–2 Human Development

People develop physically, intellectually, emotionally, and socially. These types of development are related and affect each other. Following are descriptions of the types of human development:

- **Physical development** is the growth and change of the body. Other types of human development build on these physical changes. For instance, the brain develops and grows more complex in structure. These changes allow a person to learn and think in more complex ways.

- **Intellectual development** describes the growth of a person's ability to think, learn, and respond to the world. It includes learning to communicate, including using sign language, reading Braille, speaking, reading, and writing.
- **Emotional development** is the formation of a person's identity, personality, independence, and self-esteem.
- **Social development** describes the ability to interact with others in positive ways. Social skills develop throughout a person's life.

Influences on Development

Many factors affect how a person develops (**Figure 8.1.3**). A person's genetic makeup affects how a person develops. Genes are inherited from a person's biological parents. Each person's genetic makeup is unique, except in the case of identical twins.

A person's genetic makeup sets certain physical traits, such as hair and eye color. It influences other traits, such as a person's height. However, height is also affected by other factors, such as the food a child eats or childhood illness.

The environment a person lives in affects how they develop. Growing up in a small town is different from growing up in a large city. Another important part of a person's environment is their access to quality healthcare. These different experiences and conditions can affect how a child develops.

The decisions that a person makes have a major impact on development. When people are young, the decisions that their parents or guardians make on their behalf can also impact their development. For example, introducing children to physical activity, healthy eating, and reading can all have an influence on how a child develops.

A person's friends can have an impact, too. Responsible, caring friends can influence a person to be that way also. Similarly, friends who make risky choices can influence people to also make unhealthy choices.

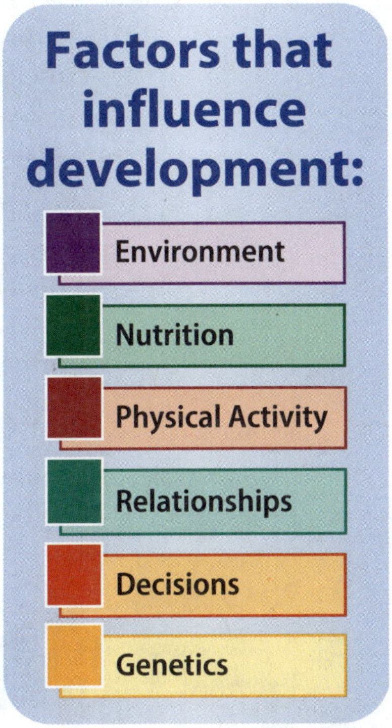

Factors that influence development:
- Environment
- Nutrition
- Physical Activity
- Relationships
- Decisions
- Genetics

Goodheart-Willcox Publisher

Figure 8.1.3 A person's physical activity, relationships, behavior, and genetic makeup are some of the factors that can affect how a person develops.

Differences in Development

People often develop in different ways. A difference in development can make it easier or more difficult for a person to perform certain tasks.

A **disability** is an example of a difference in development. Some types of disability develop before birth. Other types are caused by injuries or diseases.
- **Physical disabilities** include paralysis, loss of a limb, and vision and hearing conditions.
- **Intellectual disabilities** affect learning, social behavior, communication, and self-care habits.
- **Learning disorders** interfere with the brain's ability to process, recall, and apply information (**Figure 8.1.4**).
- **Developmental disabilities** include attention-deficit hyperactivity disorder (ADHD), cerebral palsy, autism spectrum disorder, and spina bifida.

Figure 8.1.4 Learning disorders affect a person's ability to read, write, do math, and process information.

Which learning disorder affects a person's math abilities?

Learning Disorder	Causes Difficulty with...
Dyslexia	Reading, writing, identifying words, spelling, forming sentences, and recognizing parts of words
Dyscalculia	Ordering numbers correctly; performing basic math calculations; understanding concepts like time, measurement, or estimation
Processing disorders	Making sense of sensory data (can be visual or auditory)

Goodheart-Willcox Publisher

People can learn skills and use services that help them adapt to life with a disability. Examples include Braille resources, medications, and specialized methods for learning.

Respecting Differences

Part of advocating for health is respecting the differences between people. This means respecting differences in race, nationality, sex, beliefs, and development.

Keep an open mind about all groups of people. Challenge any stereotypes or negative beliefs you or others may have. Promote respect by treating others fairly and kindly. Intervene if you see others showing disrespect.

You can advocate for people with different abilities. For example, if you know someone with limited mobility, you can help them run errands or offer to be a walking buddy.

8.1-2 Reading Checkpoint

1. List each type of development and provide an example of how you have developed so far in your life.
2. Choose at least two factors that influence development and discuss how these factors have influenced your development so far in your life.

8.1-3 The End of Life

Essential Idea

Death is the end of the human life cycle. Grief is a normal emotional response to loss or the death of loved ones.

The human life cycle ends in death. Death can be sudden, or it can be expected after a long illness. When it is expected, a person may receive **hospice care** in the time leading up to death. The goal of hospice care is to give comfort to people who are dying and their families. During hospice care, patients receive pain relief, emotional support, and comfort.

The end of the human life cycle often causes grief. The elements of grief include intense feelings of sadness and loss. A grieving person has many feelings following the death of a family member, spouse, or friend (**Figure 8.1.5**).

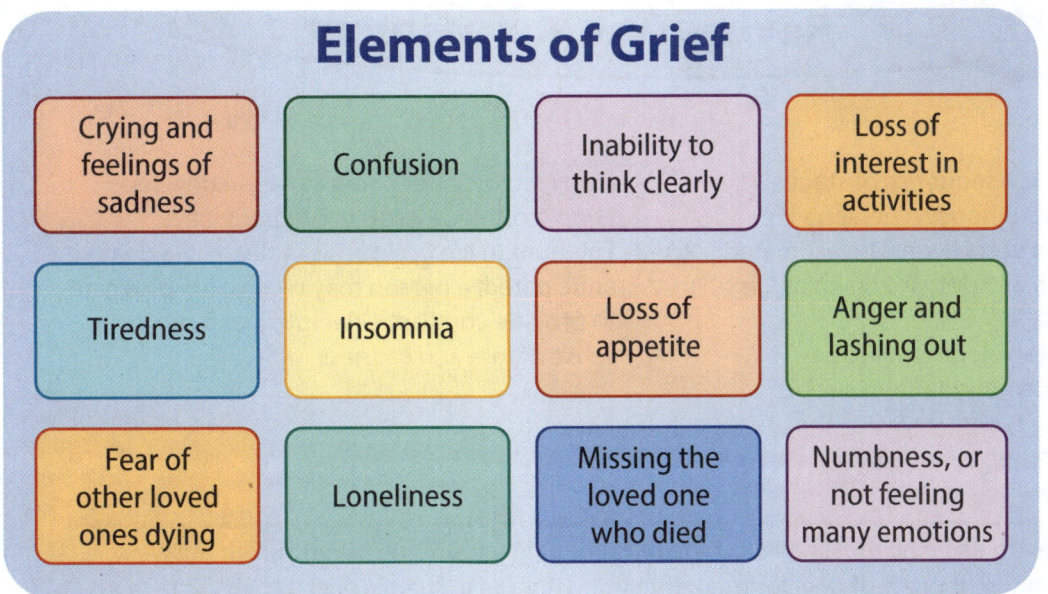

Figure 8.1.5 When a loved one dies, it is normal to feel grief. Not everyone feels all of these elements of grief.

People should grieve in the way they feel is right. They might feel very sad and cry for a long time. Some people have a delayed emotional response to a loss or death. Some might mark the loss with a ritual, such as a funeral.

Unhealthy behaviors like isolating yourself and not getting enough sleep can make grief worse. When grieving, people can practice the following healthy behaviors:

- Share feelings with trusted people. Create opportunities to spend time with friends and loved ones. Avoid spending too much time alone.
- Try to wait to make difficult decisions or major life changes until your grief decreases. If you need to make major decisions, do so with the help of close family members.
- Seek help with personal care tasks. Get professional help for coping, if necessary. Not getting necessary help can lead to depression.
- Get good nutrition, physical activity, and adequate sleep.

8.1-3 Reading Checkpoint

1. What emotions might a grieving person feel?
2. Name three healthy ways a person can grieve when they lose a loved one.

Lesson 8.1 Review and Assessment

Reading Summary

8.1–1 The human life cycle is a sequence of stages from birth through adulthood. A person's life span is the number of years lived. The estimated life span for people in a society is known as life expectancy.

8.1–2 The types of human development include physical, intellectual, emotional, and social. Many factors affect how a person develops. People often develop in different ways.

8.1–3 The human life cycle ends in death. If a death is anticipated, a person may receive hospice care to provide comfort. Grief involves a profound sense of loss and sadness.

Critical Thinking

1. **Conclude.** What do you think is the most critical stage of human development? Defend your answer.
2. **Explore.** How do the different types of development interact with and influence each other?

Develop Your Skills

1. **Communicate with Others.** Talk with your parents, guardians, or other trusted adults about your childhood, from infancy through your middle childhood years. Ask about all parts of your development (physical, intellectual, emotional, and social). Combine the information from this conversation with your memories to create a timeline of your childhood so far. Use images and pictures if you can. Are there times that are harder for you to remember? What about for the adults in your life? How do your memories compare to theirs? Using appropriate verbal and nonverbal communication skills, share your timeline with a classmate or a small group.
2. **Practice Health-Enhancing Behaviors and Access Information.** Create a graphic novel or comic strip that shows a fictional person's whole life, going through each stage of human development. Doing additional research as necessary, include in each stage challenges that may be present in that stage and how healthy habits (physical, social, and mental) can help this person lead their best life.
3. **Set Goals.** Imagine that you have given yourself the following goal: *I will live until I'm 100 years old.* Considering the influences on life expectancy, write a SMART goal with several smaller goals to help you achieve this.

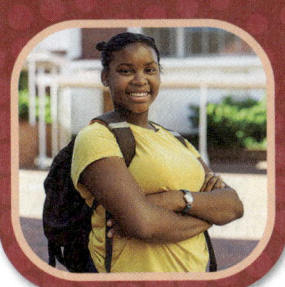

Changes During Puberty

Lesson **8.2**

Learning Outcomes

Look for the skills icon ✓ to practice health skills.
After studying this lesson, you will be able to

8.2-1 **Describe** the physical changes that occur during puberty.
8.2-2 **Summarize** the intellectual, emotional, and social growth and development that occurs during puberty.
8.2-3 **Identify** common health issues that affect young people.

Essential Question

What physical, intellectual, emotional, and social changes happen during puberty?

Reading and Notetaking Activity

On a separate sheet of paper, create a graphic organizer. As you read this lesson, take notes on each type of development that young people experience during puberty. List as many details as you can for each section of the organizer.

Physical Development

Intellectual Development

Emotional and Social Development

Goodheart-Willcox Publisher

Key Terms

puberty stage of life when the body changes as it approaches sexual maturity
menstruation discharge of some tissue and blood from the uterus
primary sexual characteristics the external and internal reproductive organs
secondary sexual characteristics features of the mature body other than the reproductive organs
growth spurt period of rapid physical growth that occurs during puberty
testosterone hormone that triggers growth and development of the male reproductive organs
estrogen hormone that triggers growth and development of the female reproductive organs

Lesson image: PeopleImages/iStock/Getty Images Plus via Getty Images

Introduction

Xavier looks forward to middle school. He hopes that he will grow taller. He is excited to play sports and make new friends. Xavier's body and mind will develop during middle childhood and adolescence. Xavier and other people his age will also go through intellectual, emotional, and social changes.

8.2-1 Physical Development

Essential Idea

During puberty, young people experience the growth of the reproductive organs. Menstruation begins. Young people complete most of their physical growth during puberty. They may develop body hair, a deeper voice, or breasts. Increased oil production may cause acne.

Physical changes are the trademark of *middle childhood* (period between 10 and 12 years of age) and *adolescence* (period between 12 and 19 years of age). During this time, young people typically complete most of their physical growth and achieve their adult height and weight. Their reproductive organs also mature, which means they become capable of sexual reproduction. **Puberty** is the period of time during which all of these physical changes are taking place.

Reproductive hormones drive the physical and emotional changes of puberty. Puberty is triggered when brain hormones affect the testes or ovaries. The testes and ovaries then release hormones that affect the development of primary and secondary sexual characteristics. **Primary sexual characteristics** are the reproductive organs. **Secondary sexual characteristics** are other features of mature bodies that appear during puberty. These may include body hair, a deep voice, or breast development (*Figure 8.2.1*).

The body goes through physical growth and many changes during puberty. Some changes occur quickly, and others happen gradually. Some young people have a **growth spurt**, in which they quickly grow taller. They may repeatedly outgrow their clothes and shoes. The growth spurt is a visible external change that occurs during puberty.

Another physical change during puberty is weight gain. Male hormones cause weight gain through muscle development. Female hormones cause

Figure 8.2.1 The body goes through physical growth and sexual maturation during puberty.

Is the growth of body hair a primary or secondary sexual characteristic?

Primary and Secondary Sexual Characteristics

Primary sexual characteristics	Secondary sexual characteristics
Males: Growth of the testes and penis; erections start to occur	**Males:** Pubic, facial, and body hair; deeper voice; broad shoulders; increased muscle mass; and more oil production on skin
Females: Growth of the ovaries, vagina, and labia; menstruation begins	**Females:** Breast development, pubic and underarm hair, widening of the hips, more body fat in hips and buttocks, and more oil production on skin

Goodheart-Willcox Publisher

weight gain through the development of body fat and muscle that are needed in the body.

Differences in Puberty Development

Young people will all experience puberty differently. It is common for the following to vary:

- when puberty starts
- when puberty ends
- rates of changes
- how much change happens

Some young people notice the signs of puberty earlier than others. Young people who look more physically mature than others can stand out. They may feel embarrassed about their differences. Young people who understand the

CASE STUDY

Akiko Feels Left Behind

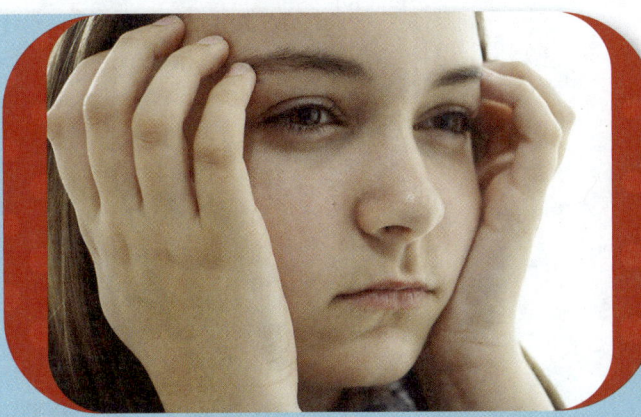

MBI/Shutterstock.com

"Why does everyone look and act so much older than me?" Akiko asks her older sister. Akiko is in eighth grade and feels like the other kids, especially the other girls, are all getting a lot taller and more mature than she is. Akiko thinks she still looks like a little kid.

There are girls in her class who have started wearing bras and shaving under their arms. Some of her friends have even gotten their periods already. Akiko feels like her body looks the same as it has for years, except maybe she is a little taller.

Akiko is not ready to be an adult yet. She likes the freedom of being a kid, but she does not want to be left behind. Some of her friends have started to ask others out on dates. There is someone Akiko thinks she likes, but she does not really know what that means. Akiko thinks maybe she just likes this person because her friends do. She might want to have a boyfriend, but she is also kind of grossed out by the idea of dating or kissing a boy.

Akiko is pretty sure she would rather just hang out with her friends, watch videos, create new and amazing food dishes, and play outside. Akiko is so confused about life right now that she does not know what she really wants. She thinks being 13 years old is tough!

 Practice Your Skills — Communicate with Others

With a partner, role-play a conversation between Akiko and her older sister. Make sure to include respect, empathy, active listening, and appropriate body language and facial expressions in your conversation. Consider the best time and place for this conversation to occur and identify it in your role-play.

changes of puberty are less likely to feel uncomfortable as their body changes. They are also more likely to have empathy for peers and friends going through these changes.

If you have questions about how your body is changing during puberty, you can ask your parents, guardians, or other trusted adults. To learn more about puberty, seek valid information. For example, you can talk to the school nurse or a doctor for accurate medical information. You can also get helpful, factual information from some websites. Choose websites carefully, though. Only visit the websites of government health agencies or valid health organizations.

Male Puberty

Male puberty often begins around 10 to 14 years of age. The hormone **testosterone** triggers growth and development of the male reproductive organs. This hormone also causes the body to form male secondary sexual characteristics. These may include pubic, facial, and body hair; broad shoulders; and increased muscle mass. The voice deepens as the larynx grows. The voice may crack as the body adjusts.

During male puberty, young people often experience the following physical and hormonal changes:

- Quick growth in height and weight. This growth rate can vary a lot from person to person.
- Oil production on the skin and scalp increases. This extra oil can lead to acne on the face, shoulders, back, and chest.
- Swelling in their breasts for some. This swelling is normal and usually goes away as puberty continues.
- Sexual feelings. Young people can become curious about sex.

As young people's reproductive systems develop, they should pay attention to possible health issues and important care procedures. They can wear equipment to protect the testes during contact sports and regularly check their testes for swelling or lumps. Young people can also see a doctor for preventive care or if they experience any signs that worry them.

Female Puberty

Female puberty often begins earlier than male puberty. The first sign of female puberty is breast development, which occurs around eight to 14 years of age. In female puberty, the hormone **estrogen** triggers growth and development of the female reproductive organs. Estrogen also causes development of female secondary sexual characteristics. These may include breast development and growth of pubic, underarm, and leg hair. During female puberty, a young person's hips widen, and fat is added to the hips and buttocks.

During female puberty, a young person's body grows quickly. They can grow up to three inches per year. By the end of female puberty, a young person may have grown 10 inches and gained 25 pounds. This growth rate may vary a lot from person to person.

Puberty: What to Expect

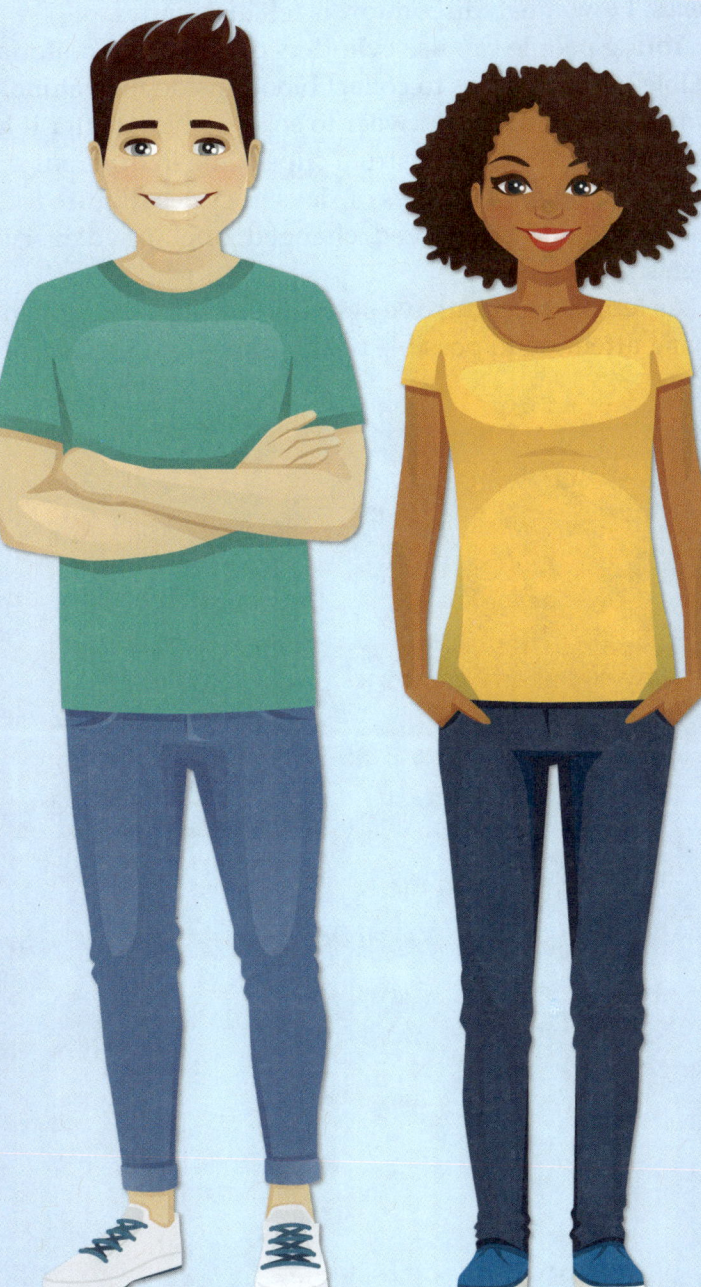

- Voice deepens, but may crack occasionally
- Shoulders broaden
- Facial, body, pubic hair growth begins
- Muscle mass increases
- Increase in height up to 4 inches per year
- Weight gain
- Acne breakouts may appear on face, shoulders, and back

- Increased oil production in skin and scalp may lead to acne
- Breasts develop
- Underarm, leg, and pubic hair growth begins
- Menstruation begins
- Increase in height up to 3 inches per year
- Weight gain and additional fat concentrated in hips, thighs, and buttocks
- Hips widen

Volhah/Shutterstock.com

Female puberty also includes the beginning of menstruation. **Menstruation** is the discharge of some blood and tissues from the uterus. The *menarche*, or first menstrual period, may be confusing and upsetting. Family members or a doctor can help a young person understand what menstruation means and how to prepare.

Each menstrual cycle lasts around 28 days. That time span can vary from person to person and even from month to month for the same person. Just before or during menstruation, a person may feel some discomfort, called *cramps*. How much discomfort is felt also varies.

Young people can use cylinders of absorbent material called *tampons* or flexible *menstrual cups* to collect blood inside the vagina. They can also place *sanitary pads* in the underwear to soak up blood after it leaves the vagina. Tampons, pads, and menstrual cups come in different sizes and absorbencies for heavier or lighter cycles or days in cycles (Figure 8.2.2). These hygiene products should be checked, changed, or emptied every three to four hours or when soaked.

As female reproductive systems develop, young people should start paying attention to possible health issues and important care procedures.

Figure 8.2.2
Depending on the heaviness of a menstrual flow, different size tampons or sanitary pads can be appropriate.

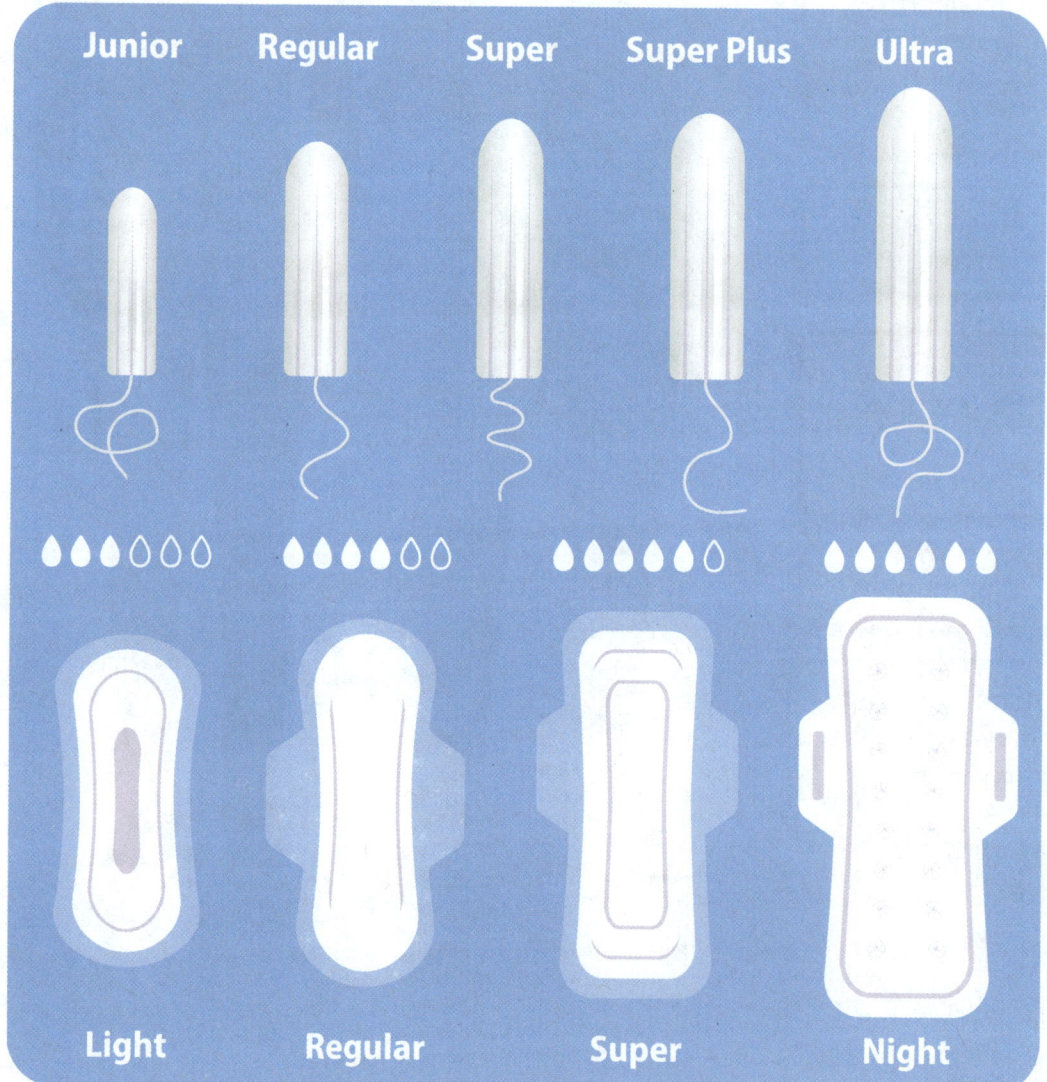

Keronn art/Shutterstock.com

Young people can change tampons and sanitary pads every four hours during menstruation and keep the reproductive area clean. Young people can also see a doctor for preventive care or if they experience any signs that worry them.

Female puberty will also cause increased oil secretion on the skin and scalp. As a result, young people may develop acne and hair may appear greasy. Alongside these physical changes, young people may experience hormonal changes that lead them to grow curious about sex.

8.2–1 Reading Checkpoint

1. Describe the changes that occur during male puberty. Include primary and secondary sexual characteristics in your description.
2. Describe the changes that occur during female puberty. Include primary and secondary sexual characteristics in your description.
3. How does the information in this section relate to middle schoolers?

8.2-2 Intellectual Development

During puberty, the brain is still developing. One of the last portions of the brain to fully mature is the prefrontal cortex (Figure 8.2.3). This brain region directs logical thinking and decision-making. The prefrontal cortex often has not fully developed until age 25.

Young people think in concrete terms, as they did in childhood. This means they often view the world in all-or-nothing terms. They may fail to see the complexity of issues. Young people may also be unable to imagine future effects of their choices. As a result, young people may act without thinking. They may take risks that can harm their health, such as using alcohol or drugs.

As young people mature, they often gain the ability to think more abstractly. This means they can see more than two sides of issues. This ability helps them think through more complex issues and understand different points of view.

Over time, some young people gain the ability to think logically about abstract concepts. Even older people, however, may fail to consider the possible effects of their choices. They can also take part in risky behaviors.

Sometimes, young people ignore what they know to be true. Instead, they may make decisions based on their emotions and social influences. For example, young people may choose to take part in risky behavior in the hopes of winning the acceptance or respect of peers. This is because their brains are still developing.

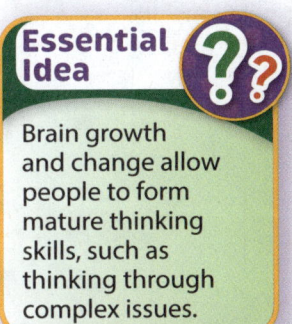

Essential Idea

Brain growth and change allow people to form mature thinking skills, such as thinking through complex issues.

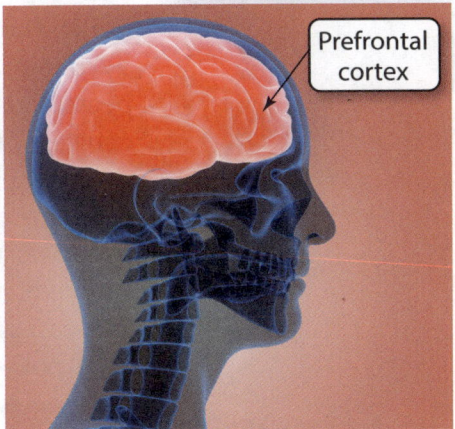

Magic mine/Shutterstock.com

Figure 8.2.3 Because the prefrontal cortex is still maturing during puberty, young people may have trouble practicing good judgment.

8.2-2 Reading Checkpoint

1. What intellectual changes occur during puberty?
2. What connections can you make between the information presented and your life?

8.2-3 Emotional and Social Development

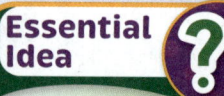

Essential Idea

During puberty, the social world of a young person may expand and become more important to them. They may seek independence from family relationships and seek new friendships or peer relationships.

Puberty comes with many developments that can feel overwhelming to some young people. New challenges and responsibilities can cause strong emotional responses. Young people may feel many emotions at once and they may find it difficult to respond calmly.

Emotional changes tend to begin earlier in female puberty than male puberty. The emotional and social changes of puberty can vary quite a lot among young people. With practice, young people can learn to manage their emotions.

Many young people want to become independent. They would like to be on their own and rely on their own judgment. Spending time with friends and joining school activities are ways to become independent. The chance to make independent choices and explore life is important for young people's social and emotional growth.

Some young people may distance themselves from their parents or guardians. They might not be as affectionate or talkative as they were as children. They may be attempting to maintain privacy and show their independence. This change can be upsetting to parents or guardians.

While some young people want to feel independent, they may still need to feel that they belong to a group. For some, their social world expands beyond family and close friends. The social world can become more important to them than it once was. Their relationships may include new friends, dating partners, teachers, and coaches. As their social life grows, young people get a taste of what adult life is like. They learn skills for maintaining social connections.

Some young people become concerned about being accepted by their peers. This means they may seek their peers' approval of their behaviors and choices. They may make decisions they think can help them fit into a group of peers. They may become self-conscious about their appearance.

Peers can be a source of support, fun, and positive peer pressure. Positive peer pressure can promote healthy behaviors. However, peers can also be a source of negative influence. Negative peer pressure is peer influence that causes a person to take part in unhealthy or risky behaviors.

Another important change in puberty is the formation of a sense of personal identity. Young people ask questions like "Who am I?" and "What am I really like?" They may act, talk, and relate to others in different ways over time. These changes are often an attempt to try out different personalities. Young people are forming the one that feels right, when they feel true to themselves. Over time, people may gain a surer sense of who they are. They can base that sense of identity on the values they hold, the goals they have, and the ways of acting that feel most right to them.

8.2–3 Reading Checkpoint

1. Describe the emotional changes that occur during puberty.
2. Describe the social changes that occur during puberty.
3. What connections can you make between the information presented and your life?

8.2-4 Health Issues in Young People

Young people face health issues that are not common in childhood or adulthood. Some of these issues arise because of newly acquired independence. For instance, having the ability to go to the mall with friends means they now face decisions about how to do so safely.

Some health issues result from new pressures from peers. Young people can be pressured to join with others in risky behaviors. Young people who think about their own identity and values can resist this kind of negative peer pressure. Thinking about the possible effects of these risky behaviors can help as well.

Using a decision-making process can help young people prepare for resisting peer pressure (Figure 8.2.4). The first step of good decision making is to identify the decision. Then you need to brainstorm options. Once you identify possible outcomes, you weigh the costs and benefits of each option. Use your values and goals to help analyze these costs and benefits. Then choose the option that has the best balance of costs and benefits for you. Taking this approach can help you resist negative peer pressure.

Other issues young people face include accidents and injuries, substance use, and mental illness. Skills for handling issues include the following:

- Learn where to find reliable health information and evaluate health information carefully.
- Remember the harmful effects of substances like nicotine, alcohol, and drugs.

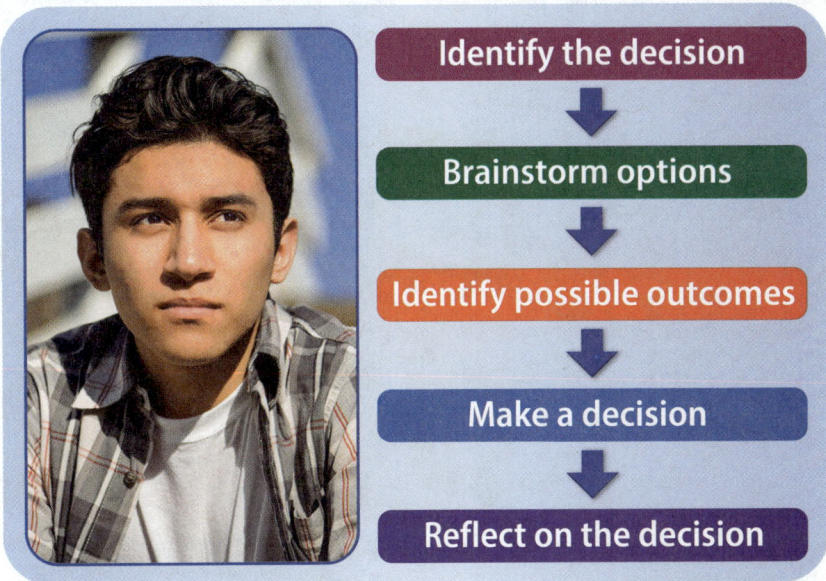

mdurson/Shutterstock.com

Figure 8.2.4 Using the decision-making process can help young people, who are learning what they think is right and wrong, stand up for their beliefs and values.

- Manage your time so you can balance school, physical activity, and fun.
- Develop healthy relationships with family, friends, and classmates.
- Ask parents or other trusted adults for help making important decisions, coping with stress, and solving issues.
- Set short- and long-term goals and make plans for achieving them.

BUILDING YOUR SKILLS — Community Connections

Peer Pressure Throughout the Life Span

During middle childhood and adolescence, peers may become a major source of positive or negative stress. Peers are people around the same age, and they have a big influence on a person's decisions, behaviors, and life, especially through middle childhood and adolescence, but even throughout adulthood.

Sometimes, peers will directly ask or tell another person to do something (external peer pressure). Other times, the pressure is internal, meaning the individual wants to do something that others are doing because they want to fit in. The desire to fit in and belong with others is a natural and powerful feeling. Both types of peer pressure (internal and external) can be positive and persuade people to do great things. Both can also be negative, however, and push people to behave in ways that do not promote physical, social, or mental and emotional health.

Practice Your Skills — Make Decisions

With a partner, create a list of decisions that young people will likely need to make throughout their middle school years. Go through this list and determine which ones are likely to involve peer pressure. For one of the peer pressure situations, determine what options a young person has and identify the pros and cons of each option. Determine which option is the best and be prepared to explain why.

8.2–4 Reading Checkpoint

1. What are some health issues young people experience? How can young people manage these issues?
2. How can poor decision-making impact the health of a young person?
3. What is your greatest concern for your peers based on your experience as a middle schooler?

Lesson 8.2 Review and Assessment

Reading Summary

8.2–1 People undergo many physical changes as they enter puberty. Some of the changes during puberty include growth in height and weight, acne, and sexual curiosity.

8.2–2 During puberty, people develop the ability to handle more complex issues.

8.2–3 Young people want to feel independent, rely on their own judgment, and maintain privacy. Social relationships become more important to them. This means that peer pressure gains influence on their choices.

8.2–4 Certain skills such as refusing peer pressure, managing time, and setting goals can help young people address health issues.

Critical Thinking

1. **Assess.** Which types of changes during puberty (physical, social, mental and emotional) are the most challenging for middle schoolers to handle? Which are the easiest? Defend your answers.
2. **Recognize.** How can middle school students prepare for the changes of puberty?

Develop Your Skills

1. **Access Information.** What are the main questions you and your peers have about puberty? What rumors have you heard that you are not sure are correct? Write your questions and then find correct answers from valid and reliable sources. Explain what makes your health information valid and reliable.
2. **Communicate with Others and Analyze Influences.** In small groups, discuss situations in which a young person is likely to face peer pressure. Be sure to discuss situations that involve positive peer pressure and negative peer pressure. Plan and perform role-plays that show how the young person healthfully handles the situations. Once you have performed your role-plays, answer the following questions:
   - What strategies are effective at dealing with peer pressure?
   - How are positive and negative peer pressure alike and different?
3. **Make Decisions.** During puberty, a person's worldview and involvement in activities often expand. To make time for everything important (friends, school, family, activities, relaxation), young people often need to prioritize. Create a scenario with a partner in which a middle schooler is being pulled in many directions or has many responsibilities and desires. Then, use a decision-making process to help this young person decide how to prioritize their activities or responsibilities. Decide which activity or responsibility is the most important. Share your scenario and your reasons for how you prioritized with another pair of students.

Lesson 8.3 Human Reproduction

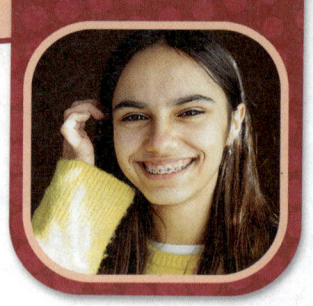

Key Terms

reproductive system body system that consists of a group of organs working together to make the creation of new life possible

ovulation release of an egg from one of the follicles into the uterus

fertilization process by which the sperm and egg combine to create a zygote

zygote egg that has been fertilized by a sperm

obstetrician/gynecologist (OB/GYN) doctor who specializes in pregnancy, labor, and delivery

prenatal development changes that occur when a zygote develops during the nine months of pregnancy

embryo mass of cells implanted in the uterus that develops for six weeks following implantation

fetus offspring that develops from the ninth week of pregnancy until birth

Learning Outcomes

Look for the skills icon ✓ to practice health skills.
After studying this lesson, you will be able to
8.3-1 **Describe** the human reproductive systems.
8.3-2 **Explain** what causes fertilization to take place.
8.3-3 **Describe** what happens during the three stages of prenatal development.

Essential Question

How does a new individual develop?

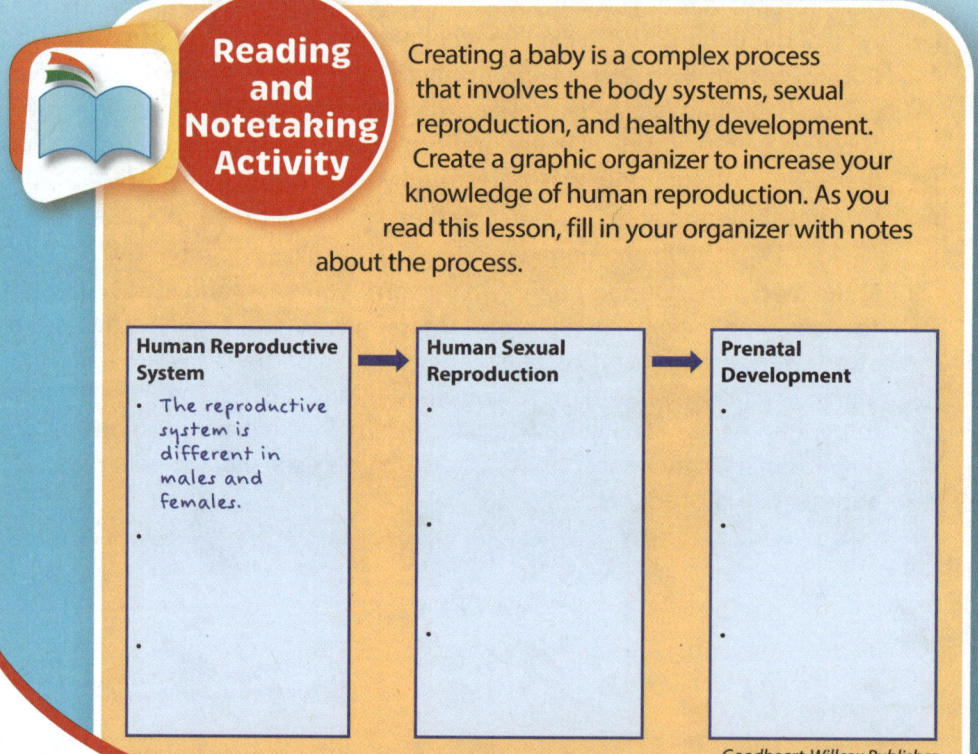

Reading and Notetaking Activity

Creating a baby is a complex process that involves the body systems, sexual reproduction, and healthy development. Create a graphic organizer to increase your knowledge of human reproduction. As you read this lesson, fill in your organizer with notes about the process.

Human Reproductive System
- The reproductive system is different in males and females.
-
-

Human Sexual Reproduction
-
-
-

Prenatal Development
-
-
-

Goodheart-Willcox Publisher

Lesson image:
asife/Shutterstock.com

Introduction

The story of Fatima's life began as a single cell. This cell was created from the merging of two cells—one cell from each biological parent. The combination of these two cells produced Fatima—a unique human being unlike any who ever has or ever will exist.

8.3-1 The Human Reproductive System

The human **reproductive system** is a body system in which organs work together to make the creation of new life possible. Unlike other body systems, the reproductive system does not begin to work until puberty. Also unlike other body systems, the reproductive system is different in males and females.

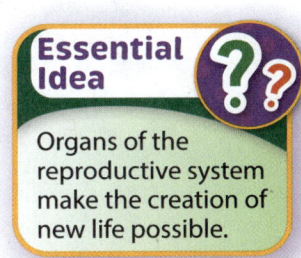

Essential Idea

Organs of the reproductive system make the creation of new life possible.

The Male Reproductive System

The organs of the male reproductive system produce and transport hormones and *sperm*, or male sex cells (**Figure 8.3.1**). Male reproductive organs include the testes and penis, seminal vesicles, bulbourethral gland, prostate, and vas deferens. These organs grow and mature as male puberty begins. The testes produce sperm and the hormone *testosterone*. The *scrotum*, a saclike structure, holds the testes.

As the sperm mature, they enter the *epididymis*. This structure is a coiled tube along the outer wall of the testes. It leads into another tube, the *vas deferens*. This tube carries sperm to the *penis*, the male organ used in sexual intercourse.

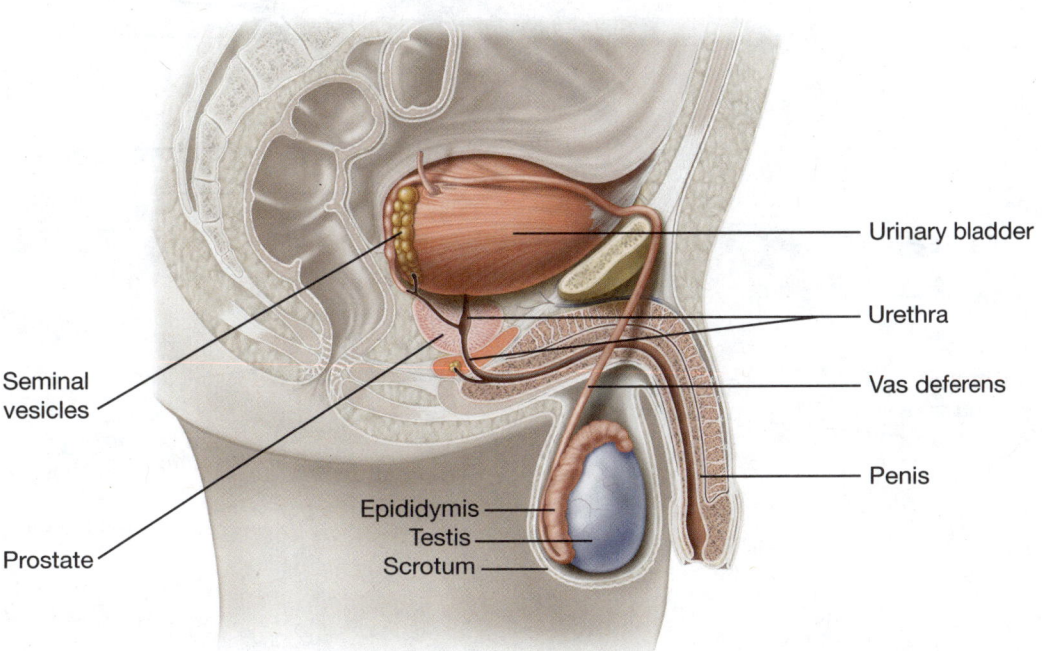

© Body Scientific International

Figure 8.3.1 This illustration shows the side view of the male reproductive organs. Sperm form in the testes (one *testis* shown) and are carried to the penis by the vas deferens. The seminal vesicles, bulbourethral gland (not shown), and prostate secrete a fluid that mixes with sperm to form semen.

The penis contains tissues that can fill with blood. When that happens, the penis becomes stiff. This is called an *erection* and happens during sexual stimulation. Intense stimulation causes the epididymis and vas deferens to contract and send sperm into the urethra. The *urethra* is a tube within the penis that has an opening at the outer end.

Before sperm leave the body, the *seminal vesicles*, *bulbourethral gland*, and *prostate* secrete fluids to form *semen*. Semen protects and nurtures sperm. *Ejaculation* occurs when more contractions force the semen out through the opening of the urethra.

The Female Reproductive System

The female reproductive organs have several functions (**Figure 8.3.2**). The *ovaries* produce female sex cells, or eggs (*ova*), and the hormones *progesterone* and *estrogen*. There are two ovaries, which are small, almond-shaped organs in the lower abdomen. Each ovary contains thousands of immature eggs. A *follicle*, which is a single layer of nurturing cells, surrounds each egg.

Starting at sexual maturity, a single egg and its follicle grow toward maturity each month. They leave the ovary and enter the nearby opening of the *fallopian tube*. One fallopian tube leads from each ovary to one side of the *uterus*. That structure is a hollow organ lined with a tissue called *endometrium*. The walls of the uterus contain strong muscles and many blood vessels. During pregnancy, a fetus develops within the uterus.

The *vagina* is a tube-like structure lined with a moist membrane. It connects to the uterus at the *cervix* and leads to an outer opening between the legs.

Figure 8.3.2 This illustration shows the side view of both the external and internal female reproductive organs.

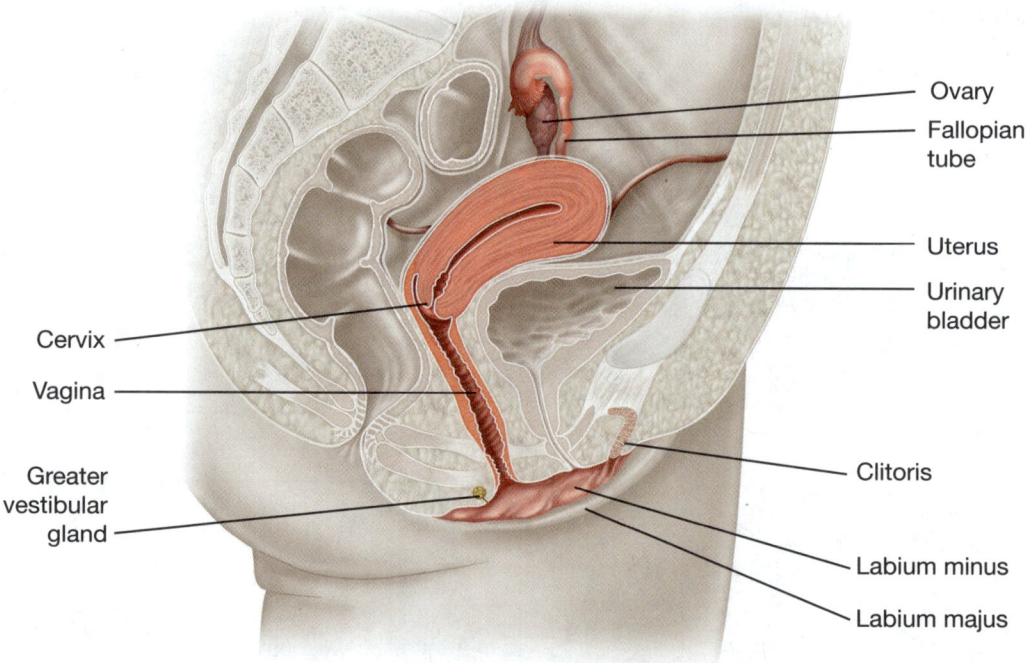

© Body Scientific International

A baby is delivered by leaving the uterus and passing through the vagina. The vaginal opening is protected by the *labia minora* and *majora* (singular *labium minus* and *majus*). Like the penis, the *clitoris* fills with blood during sexual stimulation. The *greater vestibular gland* secretes fluid to lubricate the vagina.

In female puberty, young people begin to have a menstrual cycle each month. At the start of the cycle, a follicle develops within an ovary. The follicle grows and develops with its egg. At the midpoint of the menstrual cycle, ovulation occurs.

Ovulation is the release of an egg from a follicle into the uterus. When this happens, the lining of the uterus thickens. This change prepares the uterus to accept a fertilized egg. If that does not occur, menstruation begins.

Menstruation is the discharge of some blood and tissues from the uterus (Figure 8.3.3). The amount of blood and tissues discharged varies from day to day and from person to person. It marks the end of a menstrual cycle and is followed by the beginning of a new menstrual cycle.

Monthly menstrual cycles typically start between 10 and 15 years old and stop in the late 40s or early 50s. No cycle occurs during pregnancy.

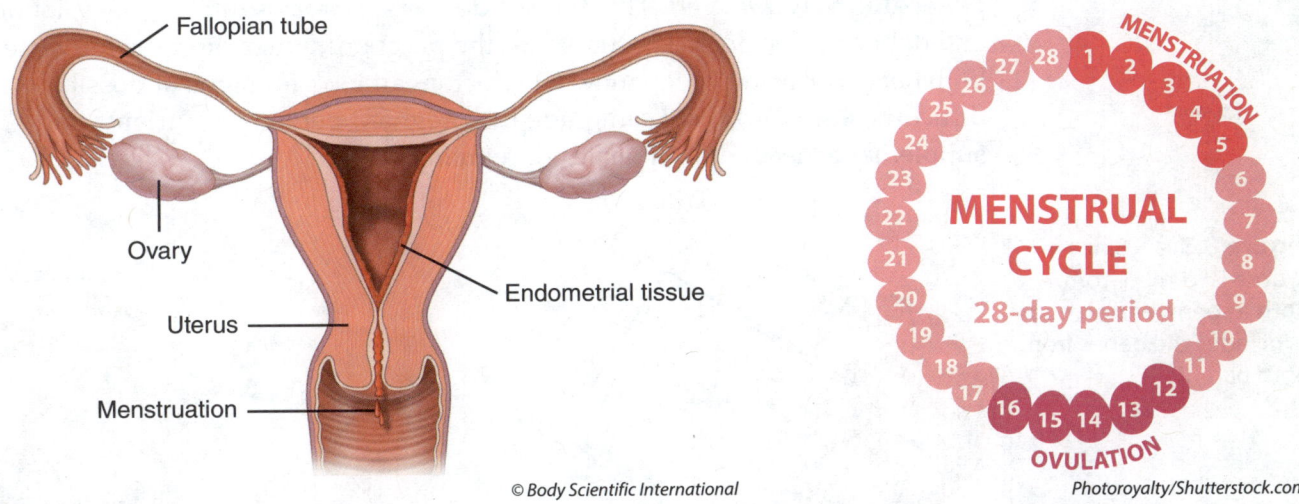

Figure 8.3.3 Eggs are produced in the ovaries and are then released into the uterus. If a pregnancy does not occur during ovulation, menstruation begins. This is the discharge of some blood and tissues from the uterus.

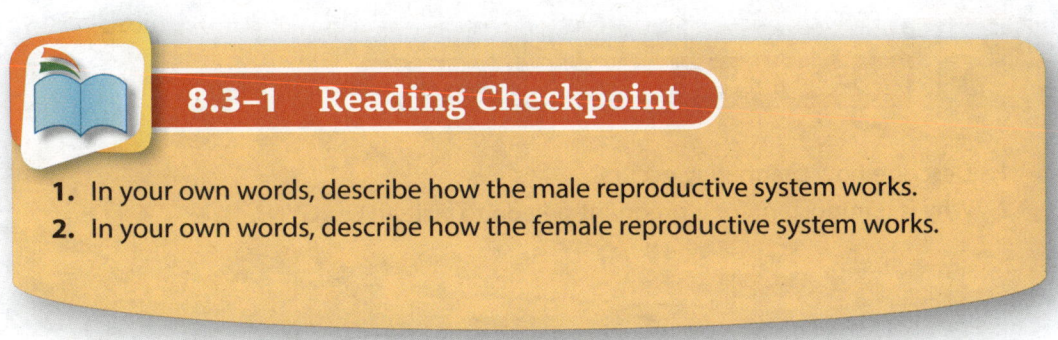

8.3–1 Reading Checkpoint

1. In your own words, describe how the male reproductive system works.
2. In your own words, describe how the female reproductive system works.

8.3-2 Human Sexual Reproduction

Essential Idea

For pregnancy to occur, sperm enters the vagina and travels to an egg in a fallopian tube. There, fertilization happens when the sperm and a mature egg combine. If this fertilized egg implants into the lining of the uterus, pregnancy begins.

Humans reproduce through sexual intercourse. For pregnancy to take place, sperm must enter the vagina. The sperm then swim from the vagina to the fallopian tube, where an egg may be located. There, one sperm and the mature egg combine in a process called **fertilization**.

When fertilization takes place, a single sperm breaks through the outer layers of the egg. The fertilized egg is called a **zygote** (Figure 8.3.4).

The zygote travels though the fallopian tube to the uterus. Inside the uterus, this ball of cells attaches to the inner lining of the uterus, a process called *implantation*. The implantation starts pregnancy by triggering the body to release hormones.

During pregnancy, the body releases hormones that stop any more eggs from being released. These hormones also prevent menstruation. Therefore, the first sign of pregnancy is often a missed menstrual period. It is important for anyone who notices signs of pregnancy to take a pregnancy test. Early testing enables a person to start prenatal care as soon as possible.

During pregnancy, people should make regular visits to an **obstetrician/gynecologist (OB/GYN)**. This type of doctor specializes in pregnancy, labor, and delivery. The doctor ensures that the pregnant person and the fetus are both healthy during pregnancy. The doctor can look for signs of possible difficulties. An OB/GYN can guide the pregnant person in nutrients and supplements needed for a healthy pregnancy.

Figure 8.3.4 Since a zygote is formed from both a sperm and an egg, it includes the genes from both parents.

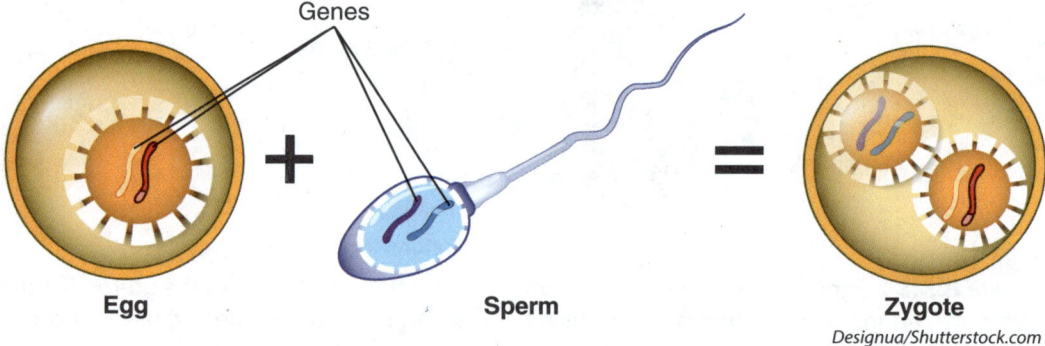

Designua/Shutterstock.com

8.3-2 Reading Checkpoint

1. Describe how pregnancy occurs.
2. Why is it important for a pregnant person to visit an OB/GYN?

CASE STUDY

Jake Learns About Reproduction

On the bus ride home from school, a few high school students were talking about how humans reproduce. Jake, a middle schooler, could not help but listen. Reproduction is something that he is curious about. He does not know much about it, and no one has really talked with him about it in detail.

The high schoolers were talking about how an influencer they follow on social media got pregnant. They were surprised that she got pregnant. They talked about a "period" and a "fertilized egg," but Jake did not know exactly what they meant. Apparently, the influencer suspected she was pregnant because of morning sickness. To confirm that she was pregnant, she then "peed on a stick."

When Jake got home, his head was spinning with the details he had just heard. He was not super familiar with all of the words they were using, even though he had heard some of them before.

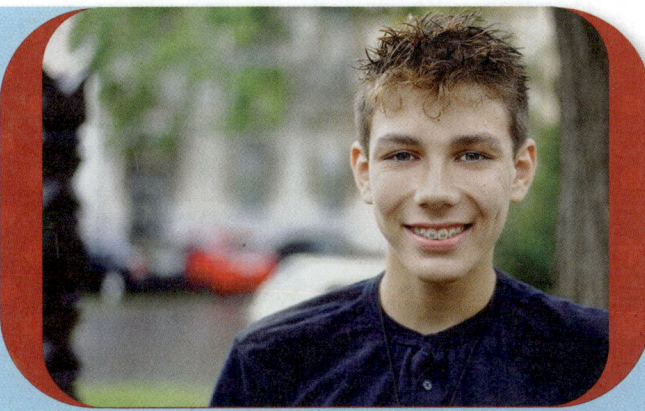
Marian Fil/Shutterstock.com

 Practice Your Skills — Access Information

To find accurate, reliable information about reproduction, Jake needs to access the right resources. Answer the following questions to understand where Jake can go for information.

1. Would you recommend that Jake ask the high school students about their conversation? Why or why not?
2. If Jake wants more information, who could provide him with accurate information about human reproduction?
3. What websites would be useful for Jake to find accurate information about human reproduction?
4. What questions do you think Jake should ask to get a better understanding of human reproduction?

8.3-3 Prenatal Development and Pregnancy

Doctors measure pregnancies in weeks. Most babies are born 36 to 40 weeks after fertilization. During a pregnancy, growth and development occur rapidly. This period of change is known as **prenatal development**. It consists of three stages.

Germinal Stage

The *germinal stage* begins with the zygote and lasts about two weeks. In this phase, the single-celled zygote divides itself into many cells. First, the single cell divides into two. These two cells then each divide, producing four cells. Those cells also divide, and so on. In five days, the zygote divides seven times, forming a ball of 128 cells. Meanwhile, this ball of cells has traveled to the uterus. After eight to ten days, it implants itself in the lining of the uterus. This implanted mass of cells is called an **embryo**.

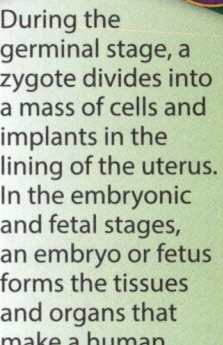

Essential Idea

During the germinal stage, a zygote divides into a mass of cells and implants in the lining of the uterus. In the embryonic and fetal stages, an embryo or fetus forms the tissues and organs that make a human.

Embryonic Stage

The *embryonic stage* lasts about six weeks. It is a critical period. During this time, the embryo begins to form the tissues and organs that make a human. Systems that will help the embryo develop also take shape during this stage (**Figure 8.3.5**). They include the following:

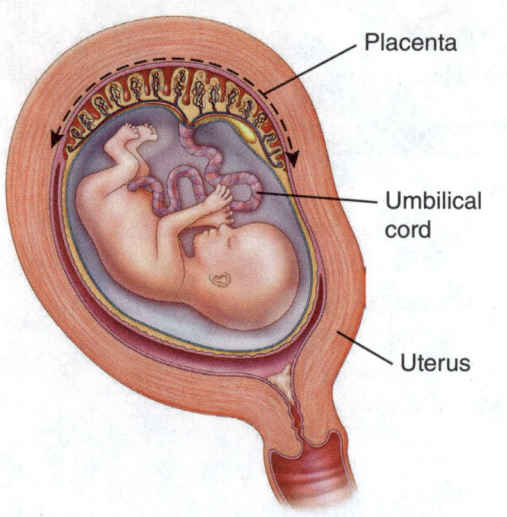

Figure 8.3.5 After the ball of cells implants itself in the lining of the uterus, the embryo begins to form the tissues and organs that make a human.

- A membrane grows and surrounds the embryo implanted in the uterus.
- An organ called the *placenta* forms in the uterus. Rich in blood vessels, it helps support the embryo. The placenta removes waste products of the embryo and supplies needed hormones to the embryo. It also prevents bacteria from reaching the embryo. The placenta blocks some—but not all—harmful substances from reaching the embryo as well. Chemicals such as alcohol, nicotine, and many drugs can still pass from the pregnant person to the embryo. The placenta cannot block them. These substances can be very harmful to the embryo.
- The *umbilical cord* also forms. This tube is full of blood vessels. It connects the placenta to the embryo at its abdomen. The cord carries food and oxygen from the pregnant person to the embryo.
- During the embryonic stage, the body's organs begin to take form. A structure called the *neural tube* forms, which will later become the brain and spinal cord. Other organs, such as the heart and liver, take on their basic shapes and organization.

Fetal Stage

The ninth week of pregnancy marks the beginning of the fetal stage. At this stage, the embryo is now called a **fetus**. This stage lasts until birth. During the fetal stage, the organs continue to grow and develop, and the fetus grows quickly. By the fourth month, the fetus has grown enough that the pregnant person looks pregnant. After nine months, most of the organs, bones, and muscles of the fetus have completed their development.

Changes During Pregnancy

The body also changes during pregnancy. Early in pregnancy, the breasts may grow larger. Skin changes during pregnancy include acne, a dark line running down the abdomen, stretch marks, pronounced moles and freckles, and darkened areolas (the area around the nipple).

Emotional changes, such as mood swings or sudden tearful outbursts, may also occur. Some side effects of pregnancy include nausea and vomiting (*morning sickness*), leg swelling, indigestion and constipation, frequent urination, backache, fatigue, and difficulty sleeping. Visits with a doctor can help people discuss these changes and detect health conditions.

Postpartum Changes and Mood Disorders

Some emotional changes continue after pregnancy ends. Temporary anxiety and mood swings can last a few weeks. People may also feel symptoms of *postpartum depression*, which is more severe and lasts longer. Postpartum depression may include the following signs and symptoms:

- feelings of unhappiness
- worry or anxiety
- exhaustion
- thoughts of harming oneself or the baby
- difficulty sleeping
- uncontrollable crying
- inability to concentrate
- difficulty making decisions

Postpartum depression is a serious health condition. This condition may not get better without treatment. If you spot these symptoms, get professional help (**Figure 8.3.6**).

Seeking Help for Postpartum Depression

- Counseling and support groups help a person recover.
- Medicine can also help a person with postpartum depression.
- Friends and family can provide emotional support and help care for the infant.
- For thoughts of harming oneself or the baby, call 911 or seek emergency help.

Goodheart-Willcox Publisher

Figure 8.3.6
Professional help and support from family and friends can help a person treat their postpartum depression.

8.3-3 Reading Checkpoint

1. Briefly describe the three stages of prenatal development.
2. What changes may occur to the body during pregnancy?
3. What can a person do if they spot symptoms of postpartum depression in a loved one?

Lesson 8.3 Review and Assessment

Reading Summary

8.3–1 The human reproductive system consists of a group of organs that begins working at puberty. Male reproductive organs include the testes and penis, seminal vesicles, bulbourethral gland, prostate, and vas deferens. Female reproductive organs include ovaries, fallopian tubes, uterus, and vagina.

8.3–2 The male reproductive organs produce and transport sperm. The female reproductive organs produce eggs. For pregnancy to occur, the sperm enters the vagina. There, one sperm and one egg form a zygote in a process called fertilization.

8.3–3 Prenatal development is the growth and development of the zygote during pregnancy. This consists of the germinal stage, embryonic stage, and fetal stage. Physical and emotional changes happen during and after pregnancy.

Critical Thinking

1. **Identify.** Which parts in the male and female body systems perform similar functions?
2. **Infer.** Why is it important for middle schoolers to learn about and understand reproductive systems and reproduction? How do you think this information can impact a person's health now and in the future?

Develop Your Skills

1. **Communicate with Others.** It can be uncomfortable to talk about reproduction, especially when using words that you do not use in everyday conversation. The best way to become more comfortable talking about human development is to practice. Using appropriate vocabulary and maturity, explain how life begins to a classmate. Start with ovulation and end with birth. After describing this process, reflect on how it felt to have this conversation and anything you could have done to make it easier or more comfortable.
2. **Advocate for Health and Communicate with Others.** Using the information in this lesson as a guide, think about when a person may need to advocate for themselves. Self-advocacy is when a person seeks help from a person or resource when they need it. Create a role-play that demonstrates someone needing help relating to human reproduction (such as understanding how it happens, prenatal care, or changes during pregnancy). Create health-enhancing messages and communication techniques for your person as the specific audience. Include in your role-play what help this person may need, who they can ask for help, and how they ask for that help.
3. **Access Information.** With a partner, use valid and reliable resources to research factors that influence the health of the fetus and pregnant person during each stage of prenatal development. Consider factors that impact physical, mental and emotional, and social health. Make a list of these factors. For each factor, list a behavior or strategy a pregnant person can do to maintain their health and the health of the fetus.

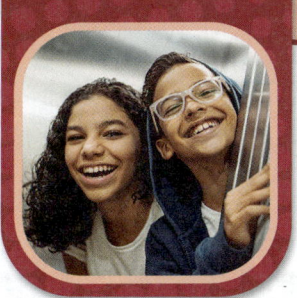

Dating Relationships and Abstinence

Lesson **8.4**

Learning Outcomes

Look for the skills icon ✓ to practice health skills.
After studying this lesson, you will be able to

- 8.4–1 **Describe** the characteristics of a healthy dating relationship.
- 8.4–2 **Examine** strategies for forming a healthy dating relationship.
- 8.4–3 **Identify** strategies to set boundaries in a dating relationship.
- 8.4–4 **Assess** the benefits of abstinence and how refusal skills can help avoid sexual activity.
- 8.4–5 **Explore** healthy ways to handle the end of a dating relationship.

Essential Question

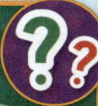

How can you form and maintain heathy dating relationships?

Key Terms

casual dating way of getting to know another person without being in a dating relationship

infatuation intense romantic feelings for another person that develop suddenly and are usually based on physical attraction

passion intense and exciting feeling based on physical attraction

exclusive committed to being romantically involved with only one dating partner

sext to send sexual content as digital text, a picture, or a video

affection expression of caring for another person

abstinence commitment to refrain from sexual activity

group dating going out with a group that includes the person one is interested in

breakup end of a dating relationship

Reading and Notetaking Activity

On a separate piece of paper, write the main headings of this lesson in the left column. As you read the lesson, take notes under each heading. Then, identify the five most important concepts you learned in this lesson and write them in the right column.

Characteristics of Healthy Dating Relationships	Five Most Important Concepts I Learned
Strategies for Forming Healthy Dating Relationships	Fact 1:
	Fact 2:
Understanding Your Boundaries	Fact 3:
Abstinence	Fact 4:
The End of a Dating Relationship	Fact 5:

Goodheart-Willcox Publisher

Lesson image:
MesquitaFMS/E+ via Getty Images

Introduction

Dating relationships are a new type of relationship for many young people. The decision to begin dating is personal. Some young people are interested in dating earlier than others. They may feel attracted to a person in a romantic way and decide to act on those feelings. Some families have rules that limit dating until a certain age.

Other young people may not yet have these feelings. They may not be sure about their preferences for a dating relationship.

Casual dating is a way of getting to know another person. A couple can go on a date without being in a dating relationship. Casual dating helps you find out whether you get along with a person. It can help you learn more about yourself (Figure 8.4.1). A *dating relationship* is when two people date on a regular basis.

For example, 13-year-old Riley feels ready to start dating. Riley's 10-year-old brother Quin, however, is not yet interested in dating. Riley and Quin's parents have a family rule that they are not allowed to date until they are 15 years old. Their parents say that Riley can begin to casually date in group settings next year in high school.

8.4-1 Characteristics of Healthy Dating Relationships

All types of healthy relationships share similar qualities. These include honesty, trust, respect, safety, care, and commitment.

Healthy dating relationships also have the following qualities:

- **Attraction.** Attraction is a physical and emotional connection that draws people together. Being attracted to someone means it feels exciting to be with that person. What a person finds attractive depends on their preferences, values, and interests.

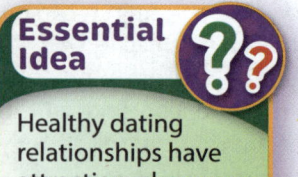

Essential Idea

Healthy dating relationships have attraction, closeness, individuality, balance, communication, honesty, respect, support, reliability, and compatibility.

Figure 8.4.1 Casual dating can help you learn more about yourself. It can also help you build interpersonal skills.

Casual Dating Is a Way to...

- learn about yourself and others
- get along with others
- form good peer relationships
- evaluate personalities
- learn about the give-and-take involved in relationships

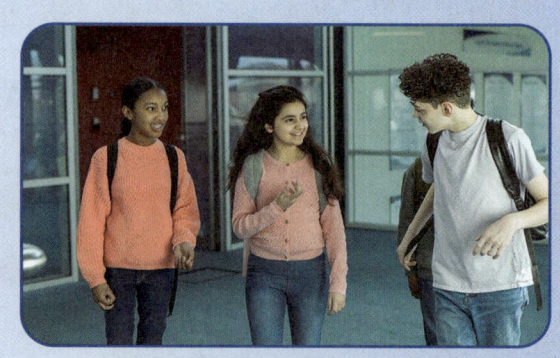

Fly View Productions/E+ via Getty Images

- **Closeness.** Closeness is when people share personal feelings and thoughts. This creates a bond. Closeness between friends is called a *platonic* relationship. If friends also share attraction, this can provide a healthy foundation for a dating relationship.
- **Individuality.** In healthy dating relationships, each person maintains their own unique identity. Their core values, beliefs, and sense of self remain the same.
- **Balance.** People in a healthy dating relationship see each other regularly, but also see friends and family members.
- **Balance of power.** Many factors, including age, race, ethnicity, gender, income, and immigration status, can affect the balance of power in a relationship. If power is balanced, each person will make decisions, choose activities, and contribute interests.
- **Communication, honesty, and respect.** People in a relationship should feel comfortable sharing their likes, dislikes, goals, values, and thoughts. They can discuss these topics openly, honestly, and with respect.
- **Support.** In a healthy dating relationship, both people support each other's successes, talents, interests, and goals. People in a healthy relationship are there for each other consistently.

Some dating relationships do not have these qualities. These relationships are unhealthy and unsafe. An unhealthy dating relationship can lead to dating violence. The signs in **Figure 8.4.2** indicate that a dating relationship is unhealthy and should end.

Signs of an Unhealthy Dating Relationship

- You feel used, ignored, and unappreciated.
- One person is more interested than the other person.
- You are subjected to angry outbursts.
- You feel you cannot say or do anything right.
- You and the other person are constantly fighting.
- You are made fun of or threatened.
- The other person is extremely jealous or controlling.
- The other person tells you to stay away from friends or family.
- The other person raises a hand as if to hit you or has ever been violent toward you.
- You are being pressured to engage in activities that make you uncomfortable.
- The other person encourages unhealthy behaviors.
- The other person does not respect your boundaries.
- One person holds more power than the other person.

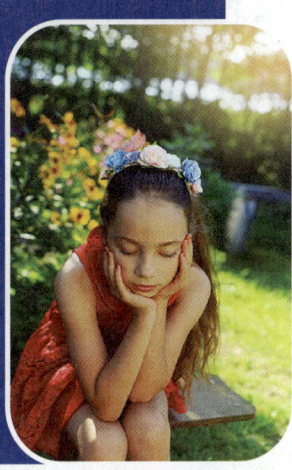

Katya Shut/Shutterstock.com

Figure 8.4.2 It can be difficult to see the signs of an unhealthy dating relationship. Talk to a parent, guardian, or other trusted adult if you see these in your relationship.

Over time, love may develop in a dating relationship. *Love* is an intense affection for and attachment to another person. Love develops gradually. It comes as people get to know each other on a deeper level and feel closer.

Love is not the same as **infatuation**. Infatuation describes intense romantic feelings that develop suddenly. It is usually based on physical attraction. Infatuation is based on **passion**. It feels intense and exciting. A *crush* is an example of infatuation.

As love develops, relationships may grow to include commitment. Sometimes commitment means promising to be **exclusive**. This means being romantically involved with only your dating partner. An exclusive couple agrees to work together on the relationship. They also work through issues when conflict occurs.

Dating can help prepare people for future marriages. Healthy marriages provide companionship. They also help people maintain social, mental, emotional, and financial health.

8.4-1 Reading Checkpoint

1. Which three qualities of a healthy dating relationship do you think are the most important? Defend your answer.
2. Explain the difference between love and infatuation.

8.4-2 Strategies for Forming Healthy Dating Relationships

Essential Idea

To form healthy relationships, get to know the person, try group dating first, cope with your nerves, and communicate with the other person.

If you are interested in dating, take steps to ensure you have a healthy relationship. Strategies include the following:

- Get to know the person. Talk to them at school, during an activity, or on the phone. This will help you find out if you share common interests and values. Take your time getting to know the person and do not rush into dating.
- Go out with a group that includes the person in whom you are interested. **Group dating** is a good way to get to know someone. Group dating reduces the pressure to keep a conversation going. It also helps you stay safe. This is especially important if you do not know the person well.
- Find ways to cope with feeling nervous. This feeling is normal. In fact, the other person will probably be nervous, too. If talking makes you nervous, plan outings that focus on an activity. You could play a game like mini golf or go to a school sporting event together.
- In a healthy dating relationship, people communicate their emotions with one another. Be open and honest about how you feel. Avoid using technology during conversations to stay present.

CASE STUDY

Martina's First Date

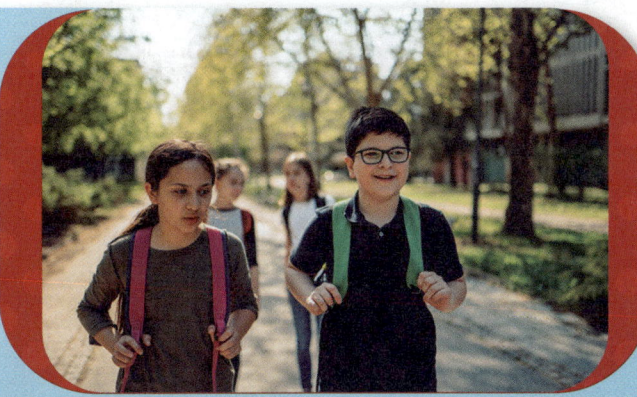
Kerkez/iStock via Getty Images

Martina was asked by Travis to go on a date. Martina finds Travis attractive. She likes his physical appearance and personality. Martina and Travis have been in some classes together. They also have some mutual friends. However, they did not know each other before this year. Martina is interested in getting to know Travis better but she is not sure if she is ready for dating.

Martina participates in many extracurricular activities. She is trying to make friends at her middle school. She worries that dating will keep her from making more friends. Martina is not sure how her parents would feel about her dating. She thinks they would accept it. According to Martina's classmates, Travis is very interested in dating Martina.

 Practice Your Skills — Communicate with Others

Imagine that Martina ultimately decides not to go on a date with Travis. Write a script for a healthy, realistic conversation in which Martina tells Travis about her decision.

8.4-2 Reading Checkpoint

1. Summarize the strategies for forming a healthy dating relationship.
2. What connections can you make between the information presented and events in the real world?

8.4-3 Understanding Your Boundaries

Dating relationships often include some type of **affection**, or ways of expressing that you care for another person. People can express affection in different ways. This could be through words, acts of kindness, or time together. For example, you can try each other's favorite activities or exchange compliments.

People can also express affection by being close to another person. This does not have to include sexual activity. Affection can mean holding hands, hugging, or sitting next to someone (**Figure 8.4.3**).

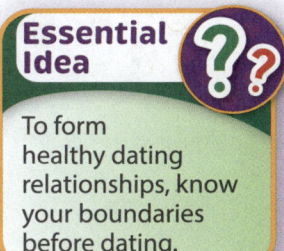

Essential Idea

To form healthy dating relationships, know your boundaries before dating.

Figure 8.4.3 You can express affection in different ways.

Some young people think you have to be physically affectionate to feel close to a dating partner. This is a **myth**.

The **truth** is... Young people can express affection and feel close without physical touch.

mixetto/E+ via Getty Images

Young people may need to have boundaries against certain activities. As young people learn more about themselves, they may be tempted or asked to **sext**, or send sexual content in the form of actual text, pictures, or videos.

Sexting has many potentially serious consequences. Legally, it can be seen as harassment and lead to lasting consequences. A person can also be charged with child pornography for sexting with a minor. Mentally and emotionally, sexting can negatively impact one's self-esteem and body image. Once sexual photos have been sent, they can be posted online or shared with others.

Before you start dating, you should know what your boundaries are. These boundaries can relate to how you express affection. However, boundaries can also relate to behaviors like how you communicate or if and how you go on individual dates. Boundaries can also relate to not sexting. Know your boundaries before you need to make a quick decision. This can help you enforce your boundaries in relationships.

Enforcing Your Boundaries

Think about your own boundaries. When you start dating, communicate these boundaries (**Figure 8.4.4**). Having healthy self-esteem and good decision-making skills helps people stick to their boundaries.

Peer pressure can positively or negatively affect people's ability to stick to their boundaries. It can also affect whether people accept and respect your boundaries. In a healthy dating relationship, people do not feel pressure to engage in any behavior. If you feel pressure to do something that is outside your boundaries, use refusal skills to reinforce your limits.

If someone sends you a sext, do not share it with others. Immediately delete the sext and tell a parent or other trusted adult. If someone asks for a sext, use refusal skills to say *no*. Remember, if someone really cares about you, that person will not pressure you.

Enforcing Your Boundaries

Decide on Your Boundaries
- Consider your values, beliefs, and goals.
- Talk with trusted adults.
- Write down your boundaries.

Communicate Your Boundaries
- Tell your partner what your boundaries are.
- Tell your partner you will enforce your boundaries.

Avoid Risky Situations
- Stay clear of situations that might compromise your boundaries.
- Leave situations that threaten your boundaries.

Act on Your Boundaries
- Clearly communicate your decision.
- Say *no* to activities that violate your boundaries.
- Repeat your decision, if necessary.
- Know that someone who loves you will respect your boundaries.

Goodheart-Willcox Publisher

Figure 8.4.4 Decide what your boundaries are before you start a dating relationship. This lets you prepare to enforce these boundaries.

What should you do in a situation that threatens your boundaries?

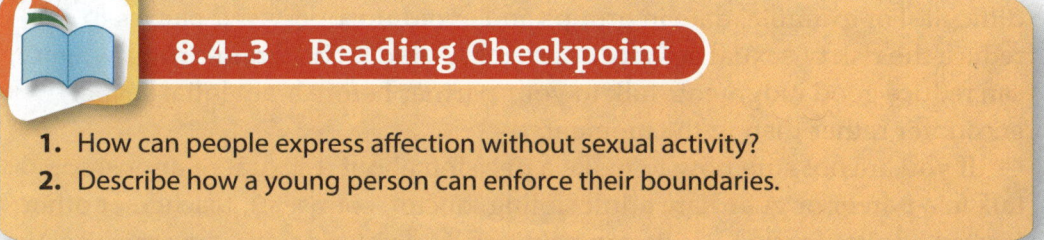

8.4-3 Reading Checkpoint

1. How can people express affection without sexual activity?
2. Describe how a young person can enforce their boundaries.

8.4-4 Abstinence

Many factors influence your decisions about affection. These include your values, beliefs, and judgment. Many young people recognize the potential consequences of sexual activity and choose *abstinence*.

Abstinence means committing to refraining from sexual activity. This is the healthiest choice for young people. Many young people have fun dating without sexual activity. Abstinence has many advantages, including the following:

- Abstinence is the only method that is 100 percent effective in preventing sexually transmitted infections (STIs), HIV/AIDS, and pregnancy.
- Sexual activity may cause intense emotions, which young people may find overwhelming. Abstinence allows young people to enjoy dating without the complications of sexual activity.
- Abstinence makes it easier for young people to focus on their individual growth, goals, and other relationships like friendships.

There are many reasons why young people choose abstinence (**Figure 8.4.5**). Knowing the reasons you want to abstain from sexual activity will help you stick to your decision.

Figure 8.4.5 Choosing abstinence allows young people to focus on their personal growth.

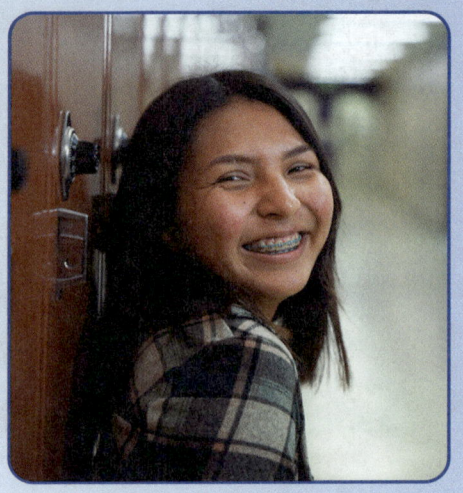

Reasons Young People Choose Abstinence

- To follow personal, moral, religious, or other beliefs and values.
- To wait until they feel ready for sexual activity.
- To wait until they find the right partner.
- To enjoy a partner's company without having to deal with the complexities of sexual activity.
- To focus on school, hobbies, or other extracurricular actvities.
- To recover from an illness, infection, or medical procedure.
- To avoid pregnancy and STIs.

grandriver/E+ via Getty Images

Supporting Abstinence

To support your decision, avoid situations that will make abstinence difficult. For example, date in groups and avoid unsupervised parties to reduce the risk of sexual activity occurring. Avoid alcohol and drugs, which can reduce good judgment. Talk to your partner before a potential sexual encounter rather than in the moment.

If you are not sure how to make a decision about a sexual relationship, talk to a parent or guardian, adult sibling, doctor, counselor, teacher, or other trusted adults. Trusted adults can help you understand your concerns so you can make a well-reasoned decision. Your decision to abstain from sexual activity is entirely your own. It is a sign of confidence and maturity to stand by your decision (Figure 8.4.6).

Talking to an adult about these matters might make some young people feel uncomfortable. The issue is too important to ignore, however. To talk effectively about these issues, choose an adult you trust. Set aside a quiet time and place to talk. Think about what you want to ask. Speak clearly and honestly about your feelings and worries. Listen fully to what your advisor has to say. You might need to have more than one talk about the subject.

iStock.com/ZouZou1

Figure 8.4.6 Abstinence from sexual activity is a sign of confidence and maturity.

Dealing with Sexual Pressure

Young people may encounter many outside pressures and conflicting messages about sexual activity. People may pressure their dating partners to have sex. Friends and peers may say that "everyone is doing it." However, most adolescents do not have sex.

Many conflicting messages about sexual activity come from the media. Advertisements, films, and other media often portray young people in sexual relationships. The implied message is that sex is a common part of adolescent relationships. In reality, millions of young people choose abstinence. In addition, media portrayals of sexual relationships often make them seem casual, with little or no risk or emotional fallout. The messages these storylines convey are not realistic.

To resist sexual pressure, remember that the actions of others are not what determine your health. Only you can make choices to promote your health and well-being. Also, practice the words and actions you would use if pressured to engage in sexual activity. Knowing what you will say or do will make dealing with sexual pressure easier (**Figure 8.4.7**). Sometimes, you may have to physically leave a situation or walk away from people who are pressuring you. Finding a group of supportive people who understand your decision to remain abstinent can also help you resist sexual pressure.

Using Refusal Skills

Refusal skills can help you respond to peer influences without going against your own goals, values, and health. Refusal skills can help when you are being pressured to do something you think is wrong, unhealthy, or against your values. With these skills, you can make independent, informed decisions.

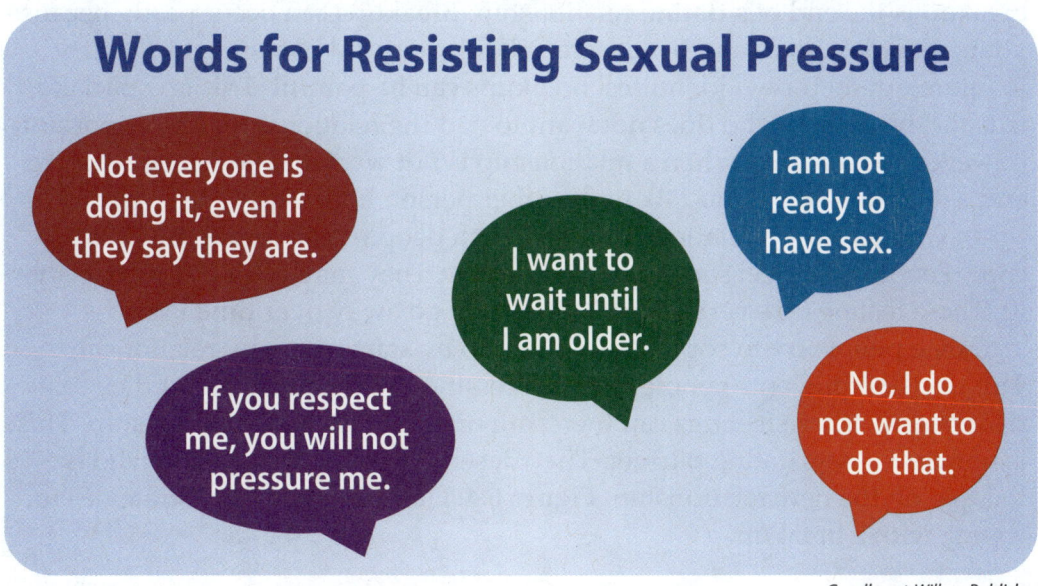

Figure 8.4.7 A great way to resist sexual pressure is by practicing what you might say in certain situations.

Goodheart-Willcox Publisher

Lesson Dating Relationships and Abstinence

Everyone has the right to refuse sexual activity at any time. The best way to refuse sexual activity is to clearly state you are not interested. Speak assertively and leave the situation, if needed. This can reduce the other person's ability to pressure you.

Partners have the responsibility to respect each other's decisions about sexual activity. If one partner does not want to engage in sexual activity, the other partner should not do or say anything that applies pressure. Partners should accept each other's decisions and avoid pressuring each other. This shows true caring and respect.

If you are being pressured to engage in sexual activity, talk to a parent, guardian, or other trusted adult for help. Negative pressure is a sign of an unhealthy relationship. You might need to end the relationship to end the pressure.

8.4-4 Reading Checkpoint

1. What are the benefits of abstinence?
2. How can you resist sexual pressure and use refusal skills to help support abstinence?

8.4-5 The End of a Dating Relationship

Many dating relationships between young people end in a **breakup.** A breakup is the end of a dating relationship. Breakups can occur partly because young people's goals and beliefs are still forming and changing as they try to figure out their own identities. Breakups can be painful. This is especially true for the person who does not want to end the relationship. It is important, however, to recognize when a relationship is not working. Someone ready to end a relationship should talk to the other person honestly.

No matter how a relationship ends, both people may find it difficult to cope. People often feel sad, angry, and lonely. They may even feel physically ill. These feelings are very normal. They will go away over time.

Some people try to cope with a breakup by starting a new relationship. This decision prevents people from processing their feelings about their last relationship. These feelings can then spill over into the new relationship. This is unfair to a new dating partner. They deserve to be with a person who is focused on the new relationship. **Figure 8.4.8** lists some healthy strategies for coping with a breakup.

Coping with the End of a Dating Relationship

- Take care of your physical and mental health
- Share your feelings with friends and family
- Keep yourself busy with activities or hobbies you enjoy
- Give your previous partner space
- Limit how much you see or hear about your previous partner
- Focus on the positives in your life

Goodheart-Willcox Publisher

Figure 8.4.8 These techniques can help you manage the end of a dating relationship.

8.4–5 Reading Checkpoint

1. In your experiences in middle school, how do young people cope with the end of a dating relationship? Are these responses healthy or unhealthy?
2. What are three healthy ways to cope with the end of a dating relationship?

Lesson 8.4 — Review and Assessment

Reading Summary

8.4–1 Healthy dating relationships include attraction, closeness, individuality, balance, open communication, honesty, respect, support, and reliability.

8.4–2 Strategies for forming healthy dating relationships include getting to know the person you want to date, dating in groups, and coping with nerves.

8.4–3 Before a dating relationship, consider your boundaries regarding affection and sexting.

8.4–4 Abstinence is the healthiest choice for young people. People can practice words and use refusal skills to maintain abstinence and avoid sexual pressure.

8.4–5 The end of a dating relationship is difficult. People need time to heal and process their feelings.

Critical Thinking

1. **Assess.** How does making and respecting boundaries promote healthy relationships? How can peer pressure and refusal skills influence boundaries?
2. **Determine.** Describe the differences between platonic friendship, infatuation, dating relationships, and marriage. What qualities are common to all of these relationships?
3. **Compare and contrast.** Compare and contrast healthy friendships and healthy dating relationships. Some people say that a healthy friendship is the foundation of a healthy dating relationship. Do you agree or disagree? Why?

Develop Your Skills

1. **Practice Health-Enhancing Behaviors.** Even if you are not yet dating, it is a good idea to think about your rights and responsibilities in a dating relationship. Reach out to a parent, guardian, or other trusted adult who has experience in healthy dating relationships to help you complete the activity. Together, answer the following questions:
   - What are my rights in the relationship? What are my responsibilities?
   - What are my partner's rights in the relationship? What are my partner's responsibilities?
   - How does respecting each other's boundaries promote a healthy relationship?
   - Should dating partners have a conversation about this information? If so, when and how should they discuss? If not, why not?
2. **Advocate for Health.** With a partner, create a "Guidebook for Dating in Middle School." Build a simple two-page guide that promotes healthy dating relationships. Use color and illustrations to make your guide visually interesting to an audience of other middle school students. Include characteristics of healthy dating relationships, ways to express affection while being abstinent, how to break up kindly, and ideas for casual and group dates in your community.
3. **Make Decisions.** Imagine that a school dance is coming up and your dating partner wants to go to the dance with you. Your friends, however, have also said that they want to hang out at the dance together. You worry about trying to make both your dating partner and your friends happy. Using a decision-making model, decide what you will do.

Module 9 Violence

Lesson 9.1 Bullying and Cyberbullying
Lesson 9.2 Unwanted Sexual Activity
Lesson 9.3 Abuse and Neglect
Lesson 9.4 Violence in the Community

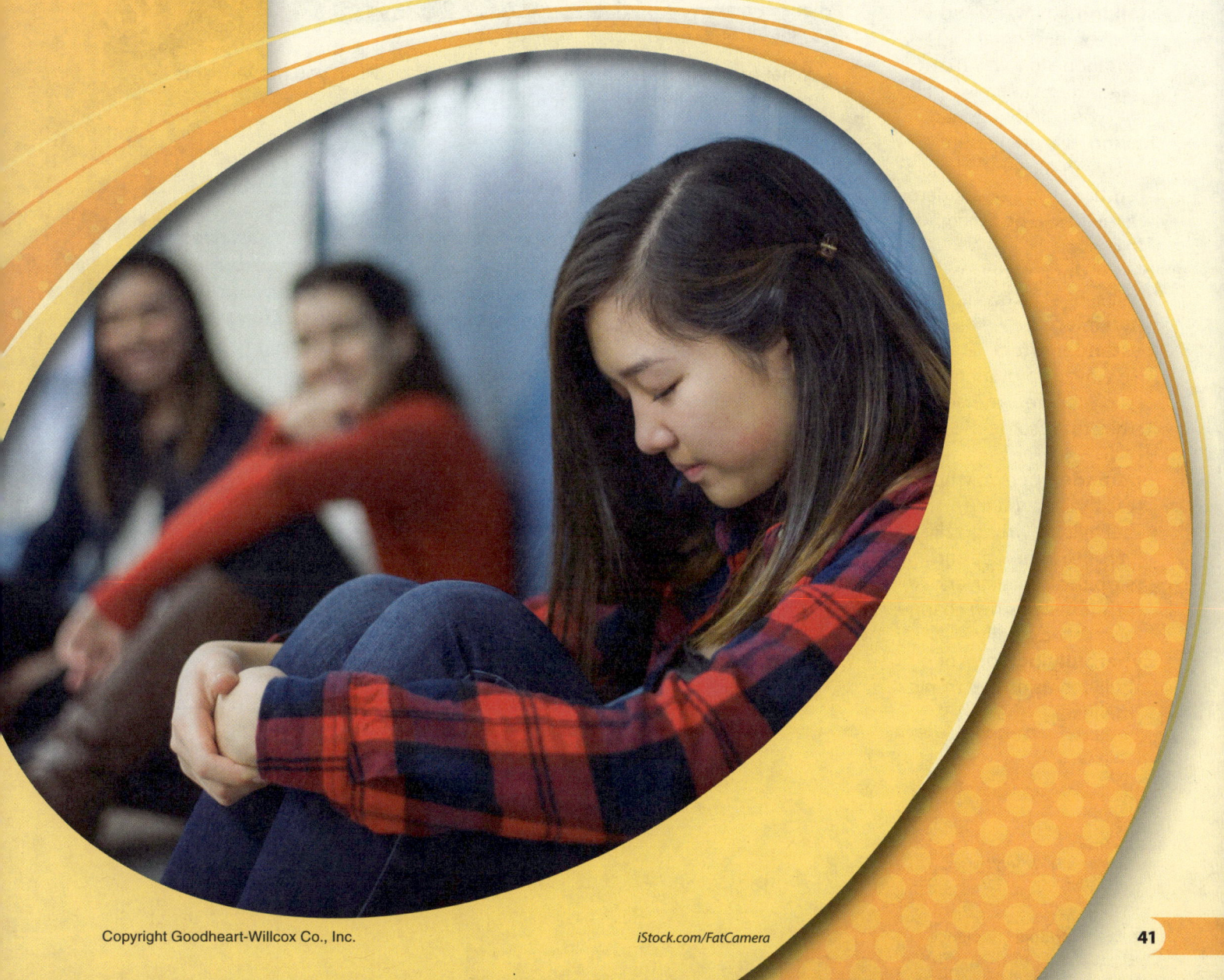

Lesson 9.1: Bullying and Cyberbullying

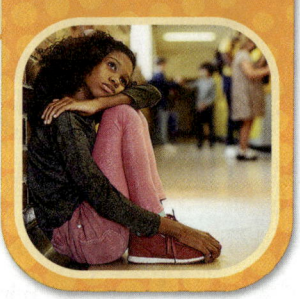

Key Terms

peer abuse violent mistreatment of one peer by another

bullying repeated aggressive behavior toward someone that causes them injury or discomfort

harassment form of bullying that targets part of someone's identity, such as race, religion, or sex

stalking following and repeatedly contacting someone in a way that leads them to feel scared, nervous, or threatened

hazing use of pressure to make someone do embarrassing or dangerous activities to be accepted by a group

bystanders people who are present at an event, but do not intervene

bystander effect situation in which a bystander is less likely to intervene because they think someone else will

upstander person who recognizes when a behavior is wrong, takes steps to intervene and stop the behavior, and promotes positive change; also called an ally

cyberbullying form of bullying using electronic means

Learning Outcomes

Look for the skills icon  to practice health skills.
After studying this lesson, you will be able to
- 9.1-1 **Explain** risk factors for violent behavior.
- 9.1-2 **Describe** the forms bullying and cyberbullying can take.
- 9.1-3 **List** the consequences of bullying and cyberbullying.
- 9.1-4 **Identify** strategies for responding to bullying and cyberbullying.
- 9.1-5 **List** strategies for bullying and cyberbullying prevention.

Essential Question

What are the consequences of bullying and how can you prevent and respond to bullying?

Reading and Notetaking Activity

In a graphic organizer, list at least five predictions of consequences of bullying and cyberbullying based on your current knowledge and experience. After reading the lesson, adjust your predictions as necessary. Then, write at least five risk factors of bullying and cyberbullying and five strategies for responding to bullying and cyberbullying.

Predictions	Risk Factors	Strategies for Responding
1.	1.	1.
2.	2.	2.
3.	3.	3.
4.	4.	4.
5.	5.	5.

Goodheart-Willcox Publisher

Lesson image: PeopleImages/iStock/Getty Images Plus via Getty Images

Introduction

Miles and Darius are brothers who go to the same school. Darius likes to play sports and is outgoing. Miles is quiet in class. Darius' friends make fun of Miles for being shy. When Darius sees them gossiping online about his brother, he feels uncomfortable.

Miles avoids many of his classmates. He feels nervous going to school. His anxiety led him to quit the school play. Miles now regrets his decision, but he does not want to spend more time with his classmates.

When you think of the word *violence*, you may not think of making fun of a classmate or spreading rumors. Both actions are examples of violent behavior.

9.1-1 What Is Violent Behavior?

Violent behavior is the intentional use of words or actions that cause or threaten to cause injury to someone or something. This includes the use of physical force, such as hitting someone, forcing someone to do something, or destroying someone's belongings.

Violent behavior can also refer to behavior that results in *psychological injury*. This means injury to a person's social or emotional health.

Many factors can lead to violence. Engaging in violent behavior, however, is a personal choice (**Figure 9.1.1**).

Violent behavior among peers may happen in schools. This mistreatment of one peer by another is called **peer abuse**. Peer abuse can include school violence and exploitation (unfair treatment of someone for personal gain) of peers. It can also take the form of bullying and cyberbullying.

In this lesson, you will learn about these types of violent behavior. You will also learn ways to respond to and prevent them.

Risk Factors for Violent Behavior

Type of Risk Factors	Examples of Risk Factors
Individual risk factors	- Lack of control over behavior and anger - History of early aggressive behavior - Exposure to violence, abuse, and conflict in the family - Use of tobacco, alcohol, or drugs - Rejection of social values or institutions - Immaturity - *Prejudice*, or unfair negative beliefs about a group of people - Discrimination and bias - Stressful events - Physical or mental health condition

Africa Studio/Shutterstock.com

Figure 9.1.1 Several factors can affect whether someone chooses violence. Risk factors do not necessarily mean that a person will act violently. Still, knowing the risk factors can prevent violence.

Which type of risk factor includes stressful events?

(Continued)

Figure 9.1.1
Continued.

Risk Factors for Violent Behavior

Type of Risk Factors	Examples of Risk Factors
Family risk factors 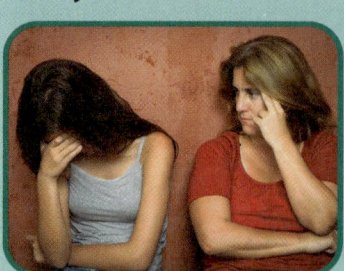 Kamira/Shutterstock.com	• Authoritarian parenting style (one that demands strict obedience) • Discipline for breaking rules that is either too harsh, lenient, or inconsistent • Poor supervision of children • Low level of involvement and emotional attachment in family • Low level of family education and income • Use of tobacco, alcohol, or drugs in the family • Criminal record • Violent behavior in the family • Access to weapons
Peer and social risk factors 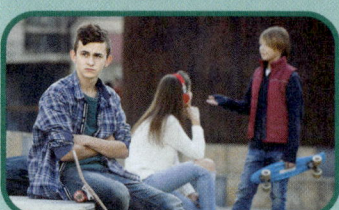 Iakov Filimonov/Shutterstock.com	• Rejection by peers • Peer pressure • Little interest or involvement in school • Involvement in gangs • Poor academic performance • Violent behavior among peers
Community risk factors 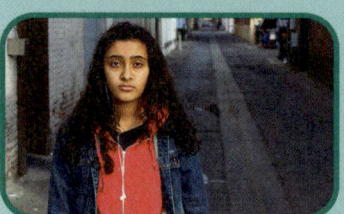 AJR_photo/Shutterstock.com	• Lack of economic opportunities • Poverty • Lack of community groups and social services • High crime and unemployment rates • Lack of healthy families in the community • High rate of families moving out of the community

9.1–1 Reading Checkpoint

1. In your own words, describe violent behavior.
2. Review the risk factors for violent behavior. List two risk factors from each category: individual, family, peer and social, and community.

9.1–2 Bullying and Cyberbullying

Bullying is repeated aggressive behavior toward someone that causes them injury or discomfort. Bullying involves using power to control or harm others (**Figure 9.1.2**).

Other forms of bullying include harassment, stalking, and hazing. **Harassment** targets someone based on part of their identity. This could be their race, religious beliefs, or sex. Harassment is a form of *discrimination*, or the unfair treatment of a certain group of people. It is illegal. Examples of harassment include

- using racial slurs
- showing symbols or words that communicate hatred toward others
- excluding or making fun of someone because of their religious beliefs, or sex

Stalking is a type of bullying that involves following and repeatedly contacting someone. This can occur in person and online. Stalking tries to control or scare someone. For example, if someone starts showing up places you visit after you say you do not want to talk, this is stalking. Stalking is a crime.

Hazing is another type of bullying. Hazing uses group pressure to make someone do embarrassing or dangerous activities to be accepted. Because it is dangerous, many states have laws against it. Hazing can include

- forcing someone to do something risky, uncomfortable, or illegal
- embarrassing someone
- making someone endure physical violence

Bullying is the fault of the person bullying others. Usually, the person bullying others has personal negative feelings or insecurities. This leads them to hurt others (**Figure 9.1.3**). Bullying is never an appropriate behavior. In fact, bullying can make a person feel even worse. It can lead to more violent behavior.

Forms of Bullying

Physical
- Hitting or shoving someone
- Cornering someone
- Pushing someone

Emotional
- Insulting or mocking someone
- Making fun of someone
- Taking someone's belongings

Social
- Spreading gossip
- Sharing someone's secrets
- Excluding someone or making them feel isolated or rejected

Goodheart-Willcox Publisher

Figure 9.1.2 Bullying can be physical, emotional, or social.

Why Does Bullying Happen?

Why Do People Bully?
- Attention
- Power
- Violent family
- History of being bullied
- Lack of sensitivity
- Low self-esteem

Why Are People Bullied?
- Age, sex, or race
- Appearance
- Interests
- Low self-esteem
- Poor social skills
- Unpopularity

Goodheart-Willcox Publisher

Figure 9.1.3 Various factors influence whether a person might bully others or experience bullying.

BUILDING YOUR SKILLS: Digital Connections

Rumor Has It

Unfortunately, rumors are a common part of young people's lives. People may spread gossip to gain popularity or status. Sometimes they spread gossip just because others are doing it.

While people can spread rumors in person, rumors spread very easily and quickly online. If one person starts a rumor in a comment or post on social media, for example, many students can share this rumor instantly.

If you have ever had a rumor spread about you, you know the pain it causes. If you have ever spread a rumor, then you probably know the uneasy feeling caused by spreading a rumor.

Gossiping is a form of bullying. So, what can you do if you hear a rumor?

- **Just STOP it.** When you hear or see a rumor, do not tell anyone else. Remember that this rumor is about a real person, and spreading this rumor will hurt that person. A rumor only lasts if people keep sharing it.
- **Do not be part of the audience.** Do not give the person spreading the rumor any attention. Instead, say, "I'm not interested in hearing mean gossip." Do not reshare posts on social media that contain rumors about other people.
- **Reverse the pressure.** Question the person who is spreading the rumor. Ask them, "How do you know this is true?" or "Is this your information to spread?" This may lead them to stop sharing this rumor.
- **Talk to the subject of the rumor.** Find a private time and place to talk to the person about whom you heard or saw a rumor. Tell them what you heard or saw. Offer to go with them to talk with a parent or other trusted adult.

Stopping the spread of rumors can feel hard. It often feels like everyone talks about other people. You can, however, be an inspiration to others. You can be the first in your group of friends, or in your school, to stop the spread of rumors.

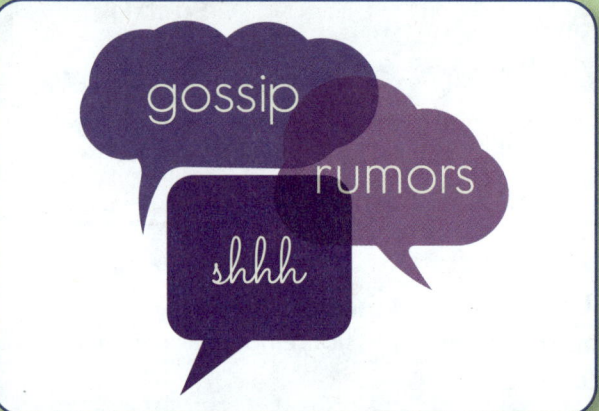

NEGOVURA/Shutterstock.com

Practice Your Skills: Communicate with Others and Practice Health-Enhancing Behaviors

Imagine a rumor was going around about someone you know. With a partner, create a realistic role-play using at least two of the strategies for responding to rumors. When selecting your strategies, consider which you are most likely to use in real life. Reflect on whether you would choose different strategies if you were alone or with a group of friends.

Cyberbullying is a form of bullying that uses electronic communication. In some ways, cyberbullying is similar to traditional bullying. Both cause emotional harm. In other ways, cyberbullying is worse than traditional bullying. Electronic communication can spread far and quickly. People can hide behind fake screen names online, which can lead them to say things they would not say in person.

Sometimes, cyberbullying happens unintentionally. One person might post a joke about someone else. They may not realize that it was hurtful. Cyberbullying that happens repeatedly, however, is not an accident. Cyberbullying can involve embarrassing, harassing, or threatening peers (**Figure 9.1.4**).

What Is Cyberbullying?

- Sending aggressive, mean, or threatening e-mails or messages
- Sharing hurtful or embarrassing messages, photos, or videos about someone on social media
- Blocking people's e-mail addresses or unfriending them on social media for no reason
- Spreading personal or embarrassing information or rumors about people
- Hacking into people's e-mail accounts or social media pages
- Impersonating others and catfishing (pretending to be someone to trick a person into a fake relationship)
- *Cyberstalking*, which can include sending inappropriate content or continuing to contact someone who does not want to talk
- Creating websites or documents to ridicule or embarrass other people

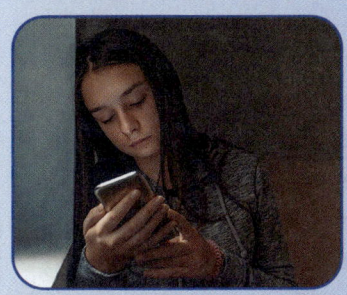

Figure 9.1.4
Cyberbullying can occur in many settings. This includes social media, texting, e-mail, chat rooms, gaming, and websites.

What is it called when a person continues to contact someone who does not want to talk?

Dragana Gordic/Shutterstock.com

9.1–2 Reading Checkpoint

1. Bullying can take many forms. Describe at least three different forms of bullying and provide an example for each.
2. Reflect on your experience with electronic communication. What are three forms of cyberbullying that have occurred or you believe could occur in your middle and high school years?

9.1-3 Consequences of Bullying and Cyberbullying

Essential Idea

Some consequences of bullying and cyberbullying include anxiety and depression, loneliness and isolation, low self-esteem, and thoughts of hurting someone or one's self. Bullying and cyberbullying can also cause changes in sleep, appetite, and behavior, anxiety about going to school or using digital devices, and withdrawal from friends or activities.

Bullying and cyberbullying can have severe and lasting consequences. Physically, people who are bullied can be injured. Bullying and cyberbullying can also cause symptoms related to stress, such as headaches, muscle pain, difficulty sleeping, and digestive conditions. Bullying and cyberbullying can lead to longer-term health conditions, such as a weaker immune system and increased risk of heart disease.

Bullying and cyberbullying can also harm a person's mental and emotional health. It can cause young people to change their behavior (**Figure 9.1.5**). It can also have serious and lasting consequences. Some of these consequences include the following:

- anxiety and depression
- fear of other people
- loneliness and isolation
- low self-esteem
- thoughts of hurting someone
- thoughts of hurting one's self

Bullying and cyberbullying also hurt the person bullying others. By bullying or cyberbullying, that person does not deal with their personal issues. They may face consequences with the law or at school. Many school districts have rules about bullying and cyberbullying. Students who bully or cyberbully others can be suspended. They can also be kicked off sports teams or other activities. Certain types of bullying and cyberbullying are even against the law. This is especially true if the behavior leads to self-harm.

People who see bullying and cyberbullying can also be hurt. People do not like seeing violent behavior. They may worry that the person will start bullying or cyberbullying them next. Bullying and cyberbullying create an environment in which stress and violence seem normal. This causes harm to everyone involved.

Figure 9.1.5 Various signs can indicate that a young person is being bullied or cyberbullied.

Signs of Bullying or Cyberbullying

- Changes in sleep, appetite, or behaviors
- Anxiety about going to school or using digital devices
- Trouble concentrating in class and on homework, which can hurt grades
- Withdrawal from hanging out with friends and family
- Withdrawal from sports or other beloved activities

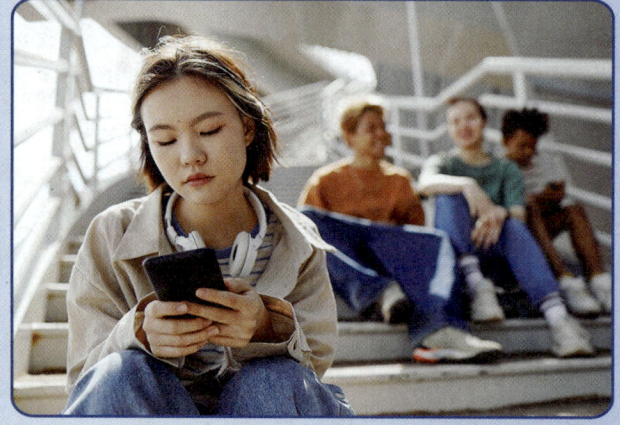

SeventyFour/iStock/Getty Images Plus via Getty Images

How to Spot Cyberbullying

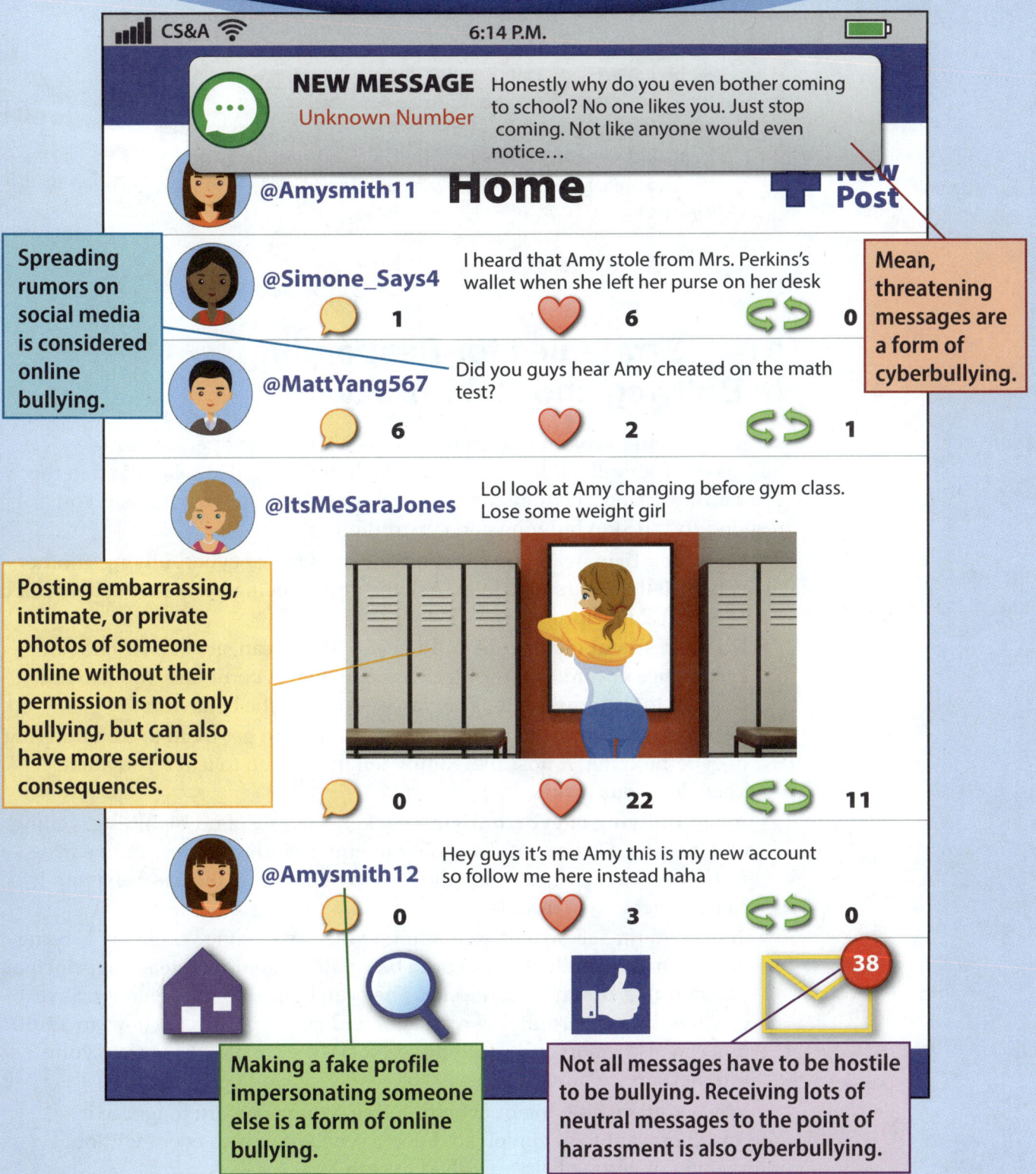

The online setting of cyberbullying makes it difficult to escape. Most young people spend a lot of time using their phones, computers, or tablets. This means cyberbullying can happen anywhere and at any time. Young people who are cyberbullied may feel they cannot escape it, even when they are at home.

9.1–3 Reading Checkpoint

1. List at least five consequences of bullying and cyberbullying.
2. How can bullying and cyberbullying also hurt people who see the violent behavior?

9.1-4 Strategies for Responding to Bullying and Cyberbullying

Bullying and cyberbullying are never the fault of the person being bullied or cyberbullied. Everyone has a right to feel safe at school and in the community. Using a combination of the following strategies can help you respond to and stop bullying and cyberbullying:

- **Do not participate.** If you see someone bullying or cyberbullying another person, tell the person to stop. Ask the person being bullied or cyberbullied how you can help.
- **Do not respond if someone bullies you.** If you can, act like you do not even notice or care. Online, block anyone who cyberbullies you. Do not respond to their messages. This can discourage the behavior.
- **Be assertive.** Simply standing up to someone can get them to stop bullying or cyberbullying. If possible, calmly tell the person to leave you alone. Then, just walk away.
- **Avoid bullying or cyberbullying back.** Do not respond by hitting, yelling, or gossiping. Do not post harassing or embarrassing content online in response. This can encourage the person to continue the bad behavior. It can also get you in trouble.
- **Tell an adult.** Talk to a trusted adult if you or someone you know is being bullied or cyberbullied. This could be a parent, guardian, teacher, principal, school nurse, or school counselor. They can help stop the behavior. Save or screenshot cyberbullying messages, videos, or photos to show an adult. You can also report cyberbullying on social media platforms or to your internet service provider.

When you see bullying or cyberbullying, you may want to ignore it. You may not want to get involved. People who witness an event without intervening or getting help are called **bystanders**.

Often, bystanders are waiting for someone else to act. They may think someone else will step up. This feeling of not having any responsibility to act is the **bystander effect**.

When bystanders stay quiet, it may seem they approve of the inappropriate behavior. This can let bullying and cyberbullying continue. Instead, be an upstander. An **upstander**, or *ally*, does something to stop wrong behavior. You communicate your disapproval of the behavior. You also help the person being hurt.

Upstanders promote positive change. An upstander might tell the person bullying others to stop. They might help the person being bullied or cyberbullied get out and find help or alert an adult (**Figure 9.1.6**).

Sometimes, young people who are cyberbullied do not want to tell anyone. They may feel embarrassed. They may also worry that their parents or guardians will take away their phones, tablets, or computers. Remember that cyberbullying is the fault of the person bullying others. It is never the fault of the person being bullied.

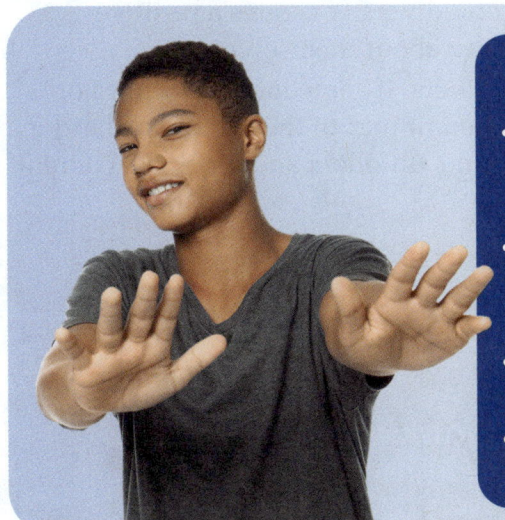

Ways to Be an Upstander

- Interrupt the situation by providing a distraction or helping the person being bullied escape.
- Tell the person bullying others to stop. Use a direct, assertive, respectful voice.
- Recruit allies by getting support from people around you.
- Support the person being bullied and assist in getting help.

Africa Studio/Shutterstock.com

Figure 9.1.6 Most middle school students think bullying and cyberbullying is a bad idea. They may not, however, speak up to stop it. You can reduce bullying and cyberbullying by being an upstander.

9.1-4 Reading Checkpoint

1. Describe what you can do to respond to and stop bullying or cyberbullying if you witness it.
2. How should you respond if you experience bullying or cyberbullying?

9.1-5 Bullying and Cyberbullying Prevention

Bullying and cyberbullying are serious issues in some schools. In addition to hurting people who are bullied or cyberbullied, it can cause stress and fear for all students. Many schools have programs to prevent bullying and cyberbullying. These programs teach students about bullying and cyberbullying and ways to respond.

You can also act on your own to prevent bullying and cyberbullying. The following strategies can help stop bullying and cyberbullying before it begins:

- Pay attention to yourself and your behaviors. This will help you recognize if you are bullying or cyberbullying others. Often, these behaviors come from people's insecurities. Address your insecurities by building self-esteem and healthy relationships. Get help if you are acting aggressively. Practice empathy for others.
- Build your confidence. People who bully or cyberbully may target people who seem insecure. Being comfortable with yourself can keep them away (Figure 9.1.7).
- Celebrate your peers' differences. Valuing diversity creates a positive environment. This helps people feel better about themselves.
- Avoid people who bully or cyberbully others. If someone who bullies or cyberbullies others is nearby, sit in a different part of the cafeteria. Hang out in a different place after school. Online, unfollow and block the content of people who cyberbully others.

Essential Idea

You can prevent bullying and cyberbullying by paying attention to your behaviors, practicing empathy, building your confidence, celebrating diversity, avoiding people who bully others, using the buddy system, never sharing passwords, and being careful about what you share online.

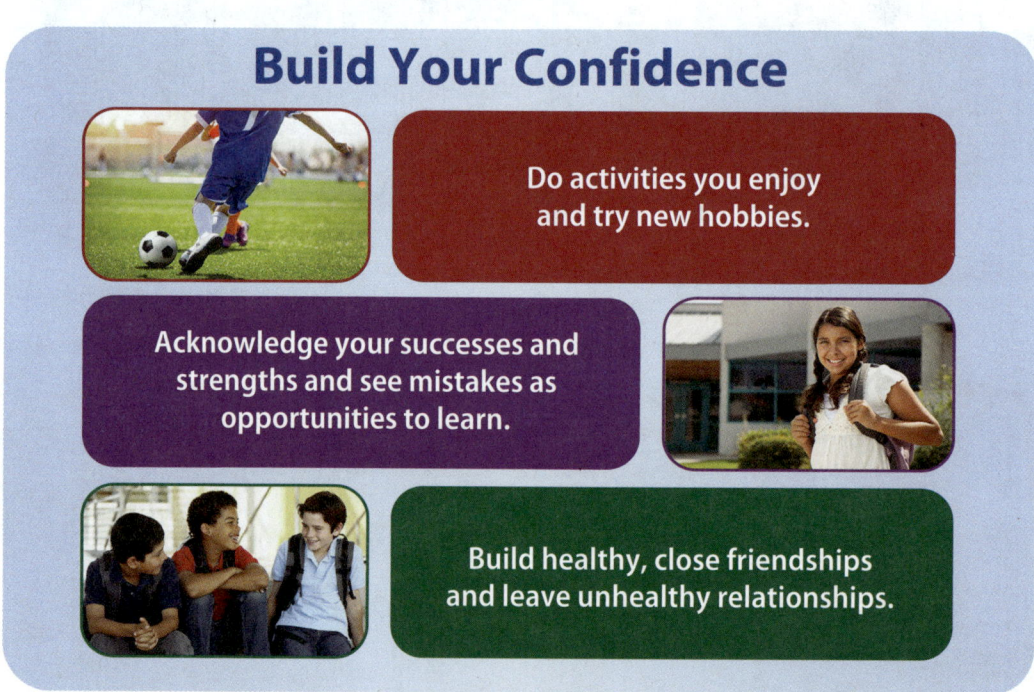

Figure 9.1.7 Building your confidence can help prevent bullying and cyberbullying.

Build Your Confidence

- Do activities you enjoy and try new hobbies.
- Acknowledge your successes and strengths and see mistakes as opportunities to learn.
- Build healthy, close friendships and leave unhealthy relationships.

Top to bottom: matimix/Shutterstock.com; Andy Dean Photography/Shutterstock.com; MBI/Shutterstock.com

- Use the buddy system. A friend can provide support if you run into someone who bullies others. People who bully others may target isolated people. Being with a buddy might prevent the person from acting.
- Increase your privacy online. Think about who can see what you post. Never share passwords to your computer, phone, or social media accounts with anyone. This prevents people from impersonating you online.
- Do not send or post anything online that you would not want shared with others (Figure 9.1.8).

If you see bullying or cyberbullying behavior at school or online, tell a parent or other trusted adult. They can help address the difficult situation and advocate for you.

Think Before You Post

- Would I say this to someone's face?
- Am I trying to get attention or make people like me?
- How would this make the person involved feel?
- Is it private? Is it *actually* private? Will it stay private?
- Do I have permission to share this?
- Will this embarrass the person involved?
- Will it hurt the reputation of the person involved?
- Could this be interpreted in a way I do not intend?
- Will I feel good about posting this later?
- Does it contain anything inappropriate?

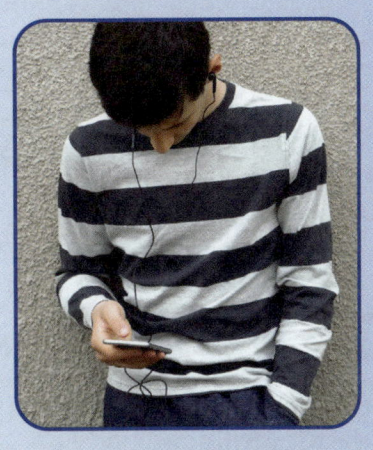

Jevanto Productions/Shutterstock.com

Figure 9.1.8 Asking these questions before you post can help you prevent cyberbullying.

9.1-5 Reading Checkpoint

1. What strategies to prevent bullying and cyberbullying do you currently use? What could you practice more? Include at least three strategies in your response.
2. How would you solve the problem of bullying and cyberbullying among middle school students?

Lesson 9.1 Review and Assessment

Reading Summary

9.1-1 Violent behavior is the intentional use of words or actions that cause or threaten to cause injury to someone or something.

9.1-2 Bullying is repeated aggressive behavior that causes physical or emotional injury or discomfort. Cyberbullying is bullying that uses electronic communication.

9.1-3 Bullying and cyberbullying can cause injuries, headaches, muscle pain, difficulty sleeping, digestive conditions, anxiety, depression, loneliness, isolation, low self-esteem, and thoughts of hurting someone or one's self. People who bully others may face consequences with the law or at school.

9.1-4 If you witness bullying or cyberbullying, be an upstander. Tell the person to stop. Avoid bullying back. Report bullying that you see or experience.

9.1-5 Schools often have bullying prevention programs. These programs teach you how to respond to and prevent bullying.

Critical Thinking

1. **Evaluate.** What role do you think teachers and school administrators have in addressing bullying and cyberbullying?
2. **Analyze.** Why are some people more at risk for being bullied than others? How can having empathy support those who are at risk for being bullied?
3. **Indicate.** If a person in your school witnesses bullying, how are they expected to respond?

Develop Your Skills

1. **Analyze Influences.** On a piece of paper, draw something you like. For example, draw your favorite animal or video game character. Then, go around a circle in small groups and describe hurtful things you have heard said in your school. For each hurtful statement, color over your drawing. Continue doing this for a few minutes. Then, as a group, discuss the following questions:
   - What did the hurtful statements your group discussed do to your drawing?
   - Can the layers of marker be taken back?
   - Would apologizing to your drawing remove the layers of marker?
   - Why do people say hurtful things to and about others?
   - How can you promote kindness toward others? Discuss the power of words, both positive and negative.
2. **Communicate with Others and Practice Health-Enhancing Behaviors.** Working in a team, plan a role-play about standing up to bullying or cyberbullying. Your role-play should resolve a conflict and use assertive communication skills. As you develop the role-play, pay attention to each team member's verbal and nonverbal communication. If someone is uncomfortable, show empathy and rework the role-play. Enlist the help of your teacher as a mediator, if needed, and perform the role-play for the class.
3. **Set Goals.** Write a SMART goal for yourself related to reducing bullying and cyberbullying. Depending on your experiences, you may write a goal from the perspective of a person who bullies others, a person who is bullied, or a bystander.

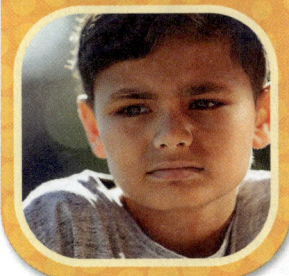

Unwanted Sexual Activity

Lesson **9.2**

Learning Outcomes

Look for the skills icon ✓ to practice health skills.
After studying this lesson, you will be able to
- 9.2–1 **Explain** the meaning of legal consent.
- 9.2–2 **Define** sexual harassment.
- 9.2–3 **Explain** how to prevent and respond to harassment.
- 9.2–4 **Describe** types and consequences of sexual assault.
- 9.2–5 **Describe** how to prevent and respond to sexual assault.

Essential Question

What steps can you take to prevent and respond to sexual harassment and assault?

Reading and Notetaking Activity

Before you read this lesson, create a graphic organizer outlining the topics in this lesson. As you read the lesson, take notes in the appropriate section. Look through the five sections after reading to review the lesson.

What Is Sexual Violence?	Sexual Harassment	Sexual Assault

Preventing and Responding to Sexual Harassment	Preventing and Responding to Sexual Assault

Goodheart-Willcox Publisher

Key Terms

sexual violence sexual behaviors that occur without legal consent

legal consent direct, verbal, freely given agreement that occurs when someone older than the legal age of consent clearly says *yes*

age of consent age at which a person can legally agree to engage in sexual activity

sexual harassment verbal or nonverbal sexual attention that occurs without legal consent

sexual assault act of threatening, pressuring, or forcing someone into sexual activity

rape sexual intercourse that occurs without legal consent

statutory rape crime that takes place when someone over the age of consent engages in sexual intercourse with someone under the age of consent

Lesson image:
courtneyk/E+ via Getty Images

Introduction

Sexual harassment and assault are serious issues. They can happen to anyone at any age. However, adolescents have a higher risk for being sexually harassed or assaulted. This is partly because their physical, emotional, and sexual development are at different levels. Some adolescents may have poor decision-making skills, increasing their risk for violence. People who are more sexually experienced may take advantage of adolescents. Sexual harassment and sexual assault are always harmful and are serious crimes.

9.2-1 What Is Sexual Violence?

> **Essential Idea**
>
> Understanding and respecting legal consent is key to preventing sexual harassment and assault. Without consent by both people, sexual behavior is sexual violence.

Sexual violence is sexual behavior that occurs without legal consent. **Legal consent** is a direct, verbal, freely given agreement that occurs when someone older than the legal **age of consent** clearly says yes. Legal age of consent varies by state. People younger than the legal age of consent cannot legally consent to sexual activity. People also cannot legally consent to engage in sexual activity if they

- feel pressured or coerced
- are under the influence of drugs or alcohol (**Figure 9.2.1**)
- have certain disabilities or disorders, such as a cognitive disability
- are asleep or unconscious

Only people over the legal age of consent can give legal consent. Legal consent does *not* occur if someone shows hesitation, does not use words, or says *no* or nothing at all. Legal consent also does not occur if someone feels pressured or coerced into saying *yes*. Agreeing to one activity or relationship does not mean a person agrees to any other activity or relationship. A person over the legal age of consent can agree to an activity and then say *no*.

Even if alcohol or other substances are present, the person who commits the sexual assault is always to blame.

Alcohol and other substances:

Reduce inhibition
- Inhibition keeps people from taking dangerous risks
- Alcohol and other substances increase the risk of dangerous behaviors

Interfere with thinking and decision-making
- Alcohol and other substances influence decision-making about boundaries, including setting and following sexual boundaries

Lessen observation skills
- Alcohol and other substances can make it harder to perceive and respect other people's boundaries

Goodheart-Willcox Publisher

Figure 9.2.1 People under the influence of alcohol, drugs, or other substances cannot legally consent to sexual activity. This is because alcohol, drugs, and other substances reduce inhibition and interfere with thinking, decision-making, and observation.

BUILDING YOUR SKILLS — Community Connections

The Importance of Consent

In certain situations, people may not consider others' feelings. When it comes to physical touch or sexual activity, people may not try to receive legal consent. Legal consent is always important, because without it, sexual behaviors are sexual violence.

1. It is essential to ask a person before any physical touch, including hugs and kisses. This question can be as simple as, "Is it okay if I…?" or "Can I…?"
2. If you do not want to give legal consent to an activity, it is important to say *no*. You do not need to explain yourself if you say *no*. Simply saying no should be enough for a person to stop.
3. Respect a person's answer. Do not do anything a person does not give legal consent to. Making them feel guilty about their answer or attempting to change their mind is not respecting their answer.
4. If a person does not respect your answer, remember to reinforce your boundaries. This can include stating your feelings confidently and walking away from a situation where your boundaries are being crossed.

Saying *no* or stating your boundaries may feel awkward, but it will feel more natural with practice.

 Practice Your Skills — **Advocate for Health**

In a small group, discuss positive strategies for setting and respecting boundaries. Brainstorm how you could raise awareness at your school of the importance of boundaries and empower students to reinforce their boundaries. Create a message that empowers middle school students. Share your message with the class. With teacher permission, share your message with others.

Certain influences can discourage discussing and respecting legal consent. The media, abusive or unhealthy relationships, and the influence of drugs or alcohol all make a person less likely to request, enforce, and respect legal consent. Healthy relationships and strong self-esteem help encourage legal consent.

Some people believe that if two people are in a romantic relationship, sexual activity cannot be violence. This is false. No one, not even a long-term romantic partner, has the right to pressure or coerce someone into sexual activity. If sexual violence occurs, the person who committed the violence is entirely to blame. The person who experienced the violence is *never* to blame. **Figure 9.2.2** lists some myths and facts about sexual violence.

Sexual violence is a serious crime, and there are laws against it. Committing sexual violence can lead to criminal charges, probation, registration as a sex offender, and time in prison. It is wrong to violate another person's boundaries or manipulate or threaten someone into sexual activity. Two types of sexual violence are sexual harassment and sexual assault. Sexual violence can also include intimate partner violence, sexual abuse, and stalking.

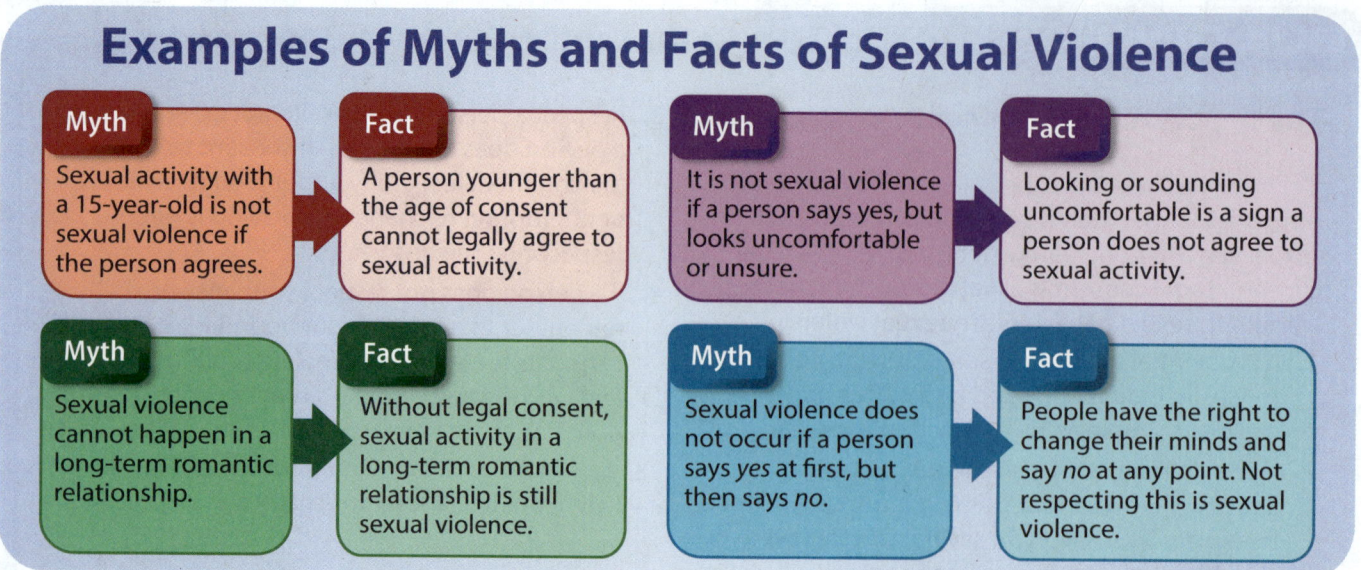

Figure 9.2.2 Knowing these facts about sexual violence can help you recognize it and get help, if needed. Sexual violence is a crime and needs to be reported to a trusted adult.

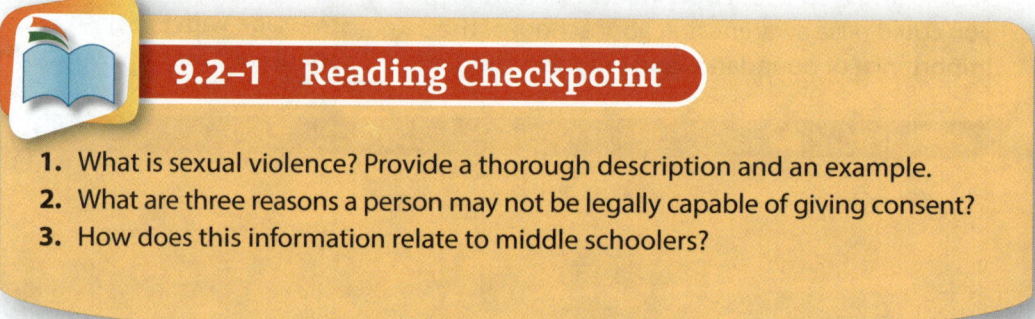

9.2–1 Reading Checkpoint

1. What is sexual violence? Provide a thorough description and an example.
2. What are three reasons a person may not be legally capable of giving consent?
3. How does this information relate to middle schoolers?

9.2–2 Sexual Harassment

As adolescents grow curious about sexual activity, they may want to talk about sex and make sexual comments. If these sexual comments are not wanted, however, it is sexual harassment. **Sexual harassment** is unwanted sexual attention, or sexual attention that occurs without legal consent. People of any sex can commit and experience sexual harassment (Figure 9.2.3).

Sexual harassment can be verbal or nonverbal. *Verbal sexual harassment* is spoken or written behavior. It can occur in person or on social media. Verbal sexual harassment can include the following harmful behaviors:

- telling sexual jokes
- spreading sexual gossip and rumors
- sexual threats
- making sexual comments to make someone uncomfortable
- pressuring someone to say *yes* after the person said *no* to a date

Nonverbal sexual harassment includes unwanted acts such as the following behaviors:

- making sexual gestures at or about someone
- making suggestive facial expressions
- pinching, rubbing, or brushing against someone in an unwanted way
- whistling at someone in a sexual way
- staring at someone's body

If you are not sure whether a behavior counts as sexual harassment, ask yourself these questions: Does it make me feel uncomfortable? Do I want the behavior to stop? If the answers to these questions are *yes*, you are experiencing sexual harassment.

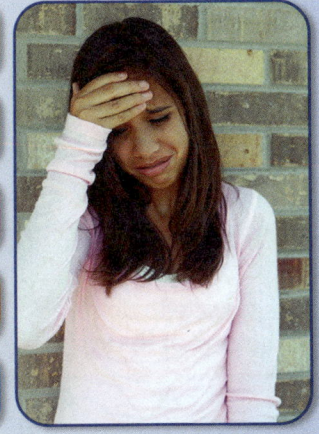

People experiencing sexual harassment can
- become **depressed**
- feel **anxious**
- lose **sleep**
- **withdraw** from normal activities
- **hate** going to school

Tracy Whiteside/Shutterstock.com

Figure 9.2.3 Unwanted sexual attention can harm a person's health and well-being.

9.2–2 Reading Checkpoint

1. What is sexual harassment? Provide a description and examples of both verbal and nonverbal forms of sexual harassment.
2. After reading this section, provide at least one question you now have or state one way this information can enhance your health or the health of others.

9.2–3 Preventing and Responding to Sexual Harassment

Communities and schools can prevent sexual harassment by teaching young people the importance of consent, promoting a culture of respect, and enforcing a sexual harassment policy.

Your behavior can also promote a culture of respect. You can be a positive role model for peers and friends. You can also discourage sexual harassment when you witness it.

To be a positive role model for friends and peers, respect their choices and their bodies. Do not pressure people to take part in harmful behaviors that others may be doing. Do not touch or hug people if you know they are uncomfortable with those interactions.

Avoid making comments or gestures that draw attention to other people's bodies. You may not know how they feel about getting this type of attention.

Essential Idea

To prevent sexual harassment, people can teach the importance of consent, promote a culture of respect, be aware of the impact of your actions, and enforce a clear sexual harassment policy. If you witness sexual harassment, be an upstander. Ask the person being harassed if they are okay or need any help.

As you learn about your friends and peers, be aware of how they prefer to interact with other people, and respect their feelings about this.

Be aware when people are uncomfortable with your behavior or the actions of others. If what you are saying or doing makes someone uncomfortable, you can change or stop your behavior. You can even show your concern by asking them if something has upset them, and apologize for your actions.

You can be an *upstander*, or ally, and intervene when you notice friends or peers being sexually harassed. It may seem scary to speak up. The good news is, most of the time, other people feel the same way you do. Others will be glad when you speak up.

An upstander can help a person being harassed by taking some simple actions. Even a comment or question from an upstander can stop the harassment.

- Ask the person if they are okay. You can tell them you see what is going on and that you do not like it either.
- Ask the person if they want the actions to stop.
- Ask the person to leave the area with you. You can say, "Let's go to the library" or "Can you help me with this homework problem?"
- Tell the person harassing someone to stop their behavior. Saying something simple is often enough to make a person stop. You can say, "Knock it off. That's gross and mean." or "I don't like what you are saying or doing to them."
- If you do not feel safe or comfortable speaking up, tell a parent, guardian, or other trusted adult what is happening. This trusted adult can also be a teacher, coach, or another school staff member. Write down details of what you saw and heard.

Young people can avoid settings that could increase the risk of being sexually harassed. This includes being alone with strangers and being where alcohol or drugs are present.

Sexual harassment is a crime. Someone who harasses others can be arrested, found guilty, and put in prison. Someone who harasses one person is likely to harass others. People who take steps to stop harassment could be helping more than just themselves (**Figure 9.2.4**).

Most schools have a sexual harassment policy. At school, people can speak with their teachers, counselors, or principal to ask for help. If you are ever sexually harassed and you are not sure what to do, talk to a parent or other trusted adult.

Stopping Sexual Harassment

- If it is safe to do so, ask the person to stop.
- Write down details of events, dates, locations, and possible witnesses.
- Print or save e-mails, pictures, videos, texts, social media posts, and other evidence.
- Report the activity to a parent or other trusted adult using the evidence.

Goodheart-Willcox Publisher

Figure 9.2.4 It can be scary to ask a person to stop harassing behavior. In these cases, try asking a friend to be with you when you confront the person. If you feel unsafe or uncomfortable, talk to a parent or other trusted adult.

9.2-3 Reading Checkpoint

1. What could you do if you witness sexual harassment to respond as an upstander?
2. How can the recommendations to prevent and respond to sexual harassment guide your behavior today and in the future?

9.2-4 Sexual Assault

Threatening or forcing someone into sexual activity is **sexual assault**. Sexual assault is a type of *sexual violence*. Sexual assault is illegal and occurs whenever there is sexual activity without legal consent.

People of any sex can commit and experience sexual assault. Those who have been sexually assaulted, including cases of rape, incest, or dating violence, are never to blame. The person committing the assault is to blame for their own actions.

Although sexual assault involves violence of a sexual nature, experts say that it is not an act of sex, but an act of power and aggression. People who commit sexual assault may use force, violence, weapons, or alcohol and drugs to make people submit to sexual acts.

Sometimes sexual assault is a form of *gender-based violence*, which targets people because of their gender. One example of a sexual assault crime is **rape**, or sexual intercourse that happens without legal consent. Sexual assault can be *aggravated* if it involves bodily injury, a weapon, or someone who cannot give legal consent. Figure 9.2.5 states additional examples of behaviors that are sexual assault.

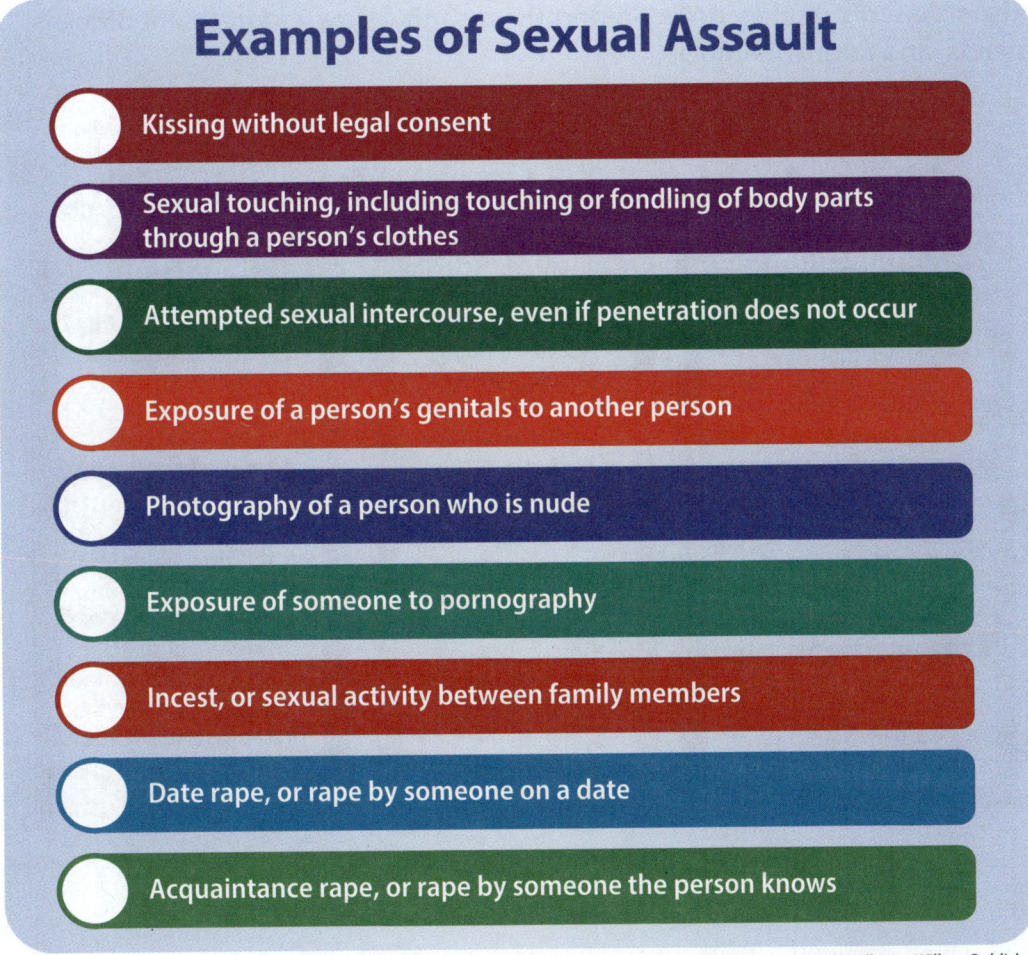

Figure 9.2.5 All of these examples are sexual assault if they occur without legal consent that is clearly and freely given.

What is it called when a person is raped by someone they know?

Goodheart-Willcox Publisher

Laws ban sexual activity between older people and adolescents who are under the age of consent. The crime of **statutory rape** occurs when someone over the age of consent has sex with someone under the age of consent. The older person can be charged with statutory rape even if the younger person agrees to have sex. For example, if the age of consent in a state is 16, a 17-year-old who has sex with a 15-year-old could be charged with statutory rape.

Sexual assault can harm the health and well-being of people who experienced the assault (**Figure 9.2.6**). Sexual assault can also have lasting and harmful effects on a person's family, friends, and community.

Some people who experience sexual assault develop post-traumatic stress disorder (PTSD). With PTSD, people may experience the following:
- repeated thoughts and flashbacks about the assault
- avoidance of anything related to the assault
- difficulty sleeping or nightmares
- irritability and jumpiness

Some people attempt to cope with the trauma of a sexual assault by engaging in risky behaviors, such as alcohol and drug use. By doing so, they increase the risk of having further health conditions. Getting professional counseling can give people healthy ways to cope with the trauma.

Though people who experience sexual assault are not to blame, some feel shame and guilt. Their self-esteem goes down, and they may withdraw from their friends and family. Many people fear blame or punishment if they tell others. As a result, they do not report the assault to law-enforcement officials, friends, and family members.

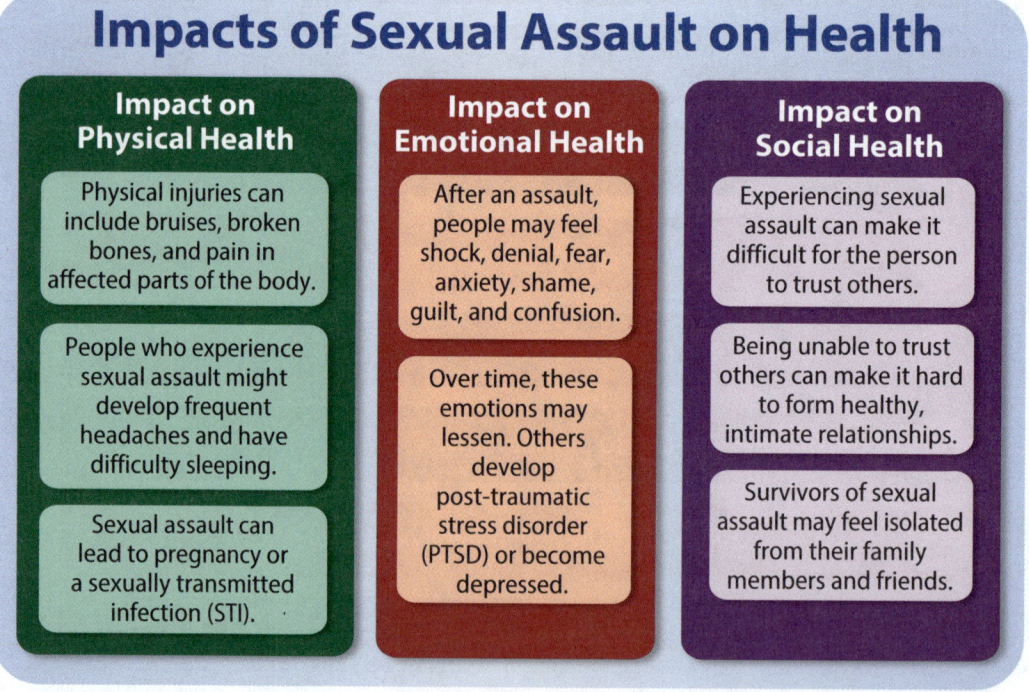

Figure 9.2.6 A person who is sexually assaulted can experience negative impacts on their physical, emotional, and social health.

Impacts of Sexual Assault on Health

Impact on Physical Health	Impact on Emotional Health	Impact on Social Health
Physical injuries can include bruises, broken bones, and pain in affected parts of the body.	After an assault, people may feel shock, denial, fear, anxiety, shame, guilt, and confusion.	Experiencing sexual assault can make it difficult for the person to trust others.
People who experience sexual assault might develop frequent headaches and have difficulty sleeping.	Over time, these emotions may lessen. Others develop post-traumatic stress disorder (PTSD) or become depressed.	Being unable to trust others can make it hard to form healthy, intimate relationships.
Sexual assault can lead to pregnancy or a sexually transmitted infection (STI).		Survivors of sexual assault may feel isolated from their family members and friends.

Goodheart-Willcox Publisher

9.2-4 Reading Checkpoint

1. What is sexual assault? Provide a definition and at least three examples.
2. Describe the effects of sexual assault on physical, emotional, and social health.
3. What is one reason sexual assault is not always reported to law enforcement officials, friends, or family members?

9.2-5 Preventing and Responding to Sexual Assault

You are in charge of your health and the decisions that promote it. Others, however, can have a powerful impact on your decisions. The best way to prevent sexual assault is to understand legal consent and treat others with respect. It is also important to know how to respond to sexual assault and support survivors.

Preventing Sexual Assault

The best way to prevent sexual assault is to learn to set boundaries and respect the boundaries of others (**Figure 9.2.7**). You can also avoid risky situations.

It is the responsibility of the person who would commit sexual assault to prevent it. People can prevent sexual assault by asking permission before touching someone else. Respect the person's boundaries by not pressuring them to do what you want.

Some situations increase the risk of sexual assault. This includes being alone with strangers or being where alcohol or drugs are present. Any time you feel uncomfortable, unsafe, or pressured, leave that situation. Call a parent, guardian, other trusted adult, or friend right away.

Essential Idea

To prevent sexual assault, understand boundaries, treat others with respect, and avoid risky situations. A person who experiences sexual assault should get medical attention right away and report the crime. Counseling and support groups can also help.

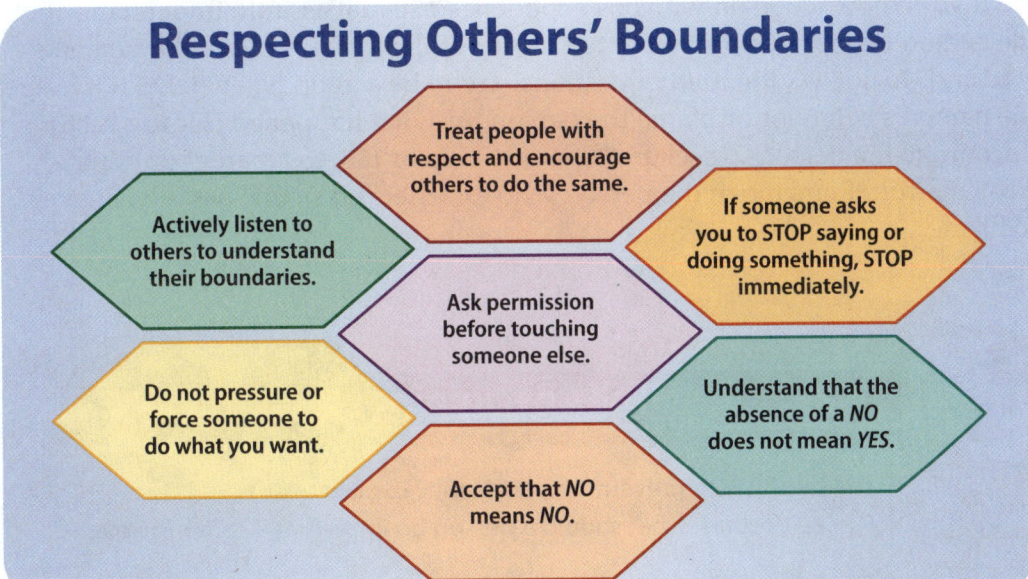

Figure 9.2.7 Making sure to respect the boundaries of others is the best way to prevent sexual assault.

What should you do if someone asks you to stop saying or doing something?

Lesson Unwanted Sexual Activity

Responding to Sexual Assault

When people experience or are threatened with sexual assault, they may experience the *fight-flight-or-freeze response*. This automatic response prepares a person's body to react to a possible danger. These reactions often cannot be controlled by the person. A person may react to the danger by fighting, fleeing, or freezing.

With a *fight* response, a person can try to fight against the danger. They may be able to scare off their attacker by struggling against them or attacking back. Physical resistance during a sexual assault can lead the person committing the assault to give up. With a *flight* response, a person can attempt to escape the danger. They can try to run away from their attackers and get help. In a *freeze* response, a person might be unable to get away or fight off the danger.

In the event of a sexual assault, a person should get to a safe place as soon as possible and call 911 or the National Sexual Assault Hotline (800-656-4673) for help. A person should also call a parent or other trusted adult. It is important to get medical attention right away at a hospital or clinic. The person will receive an examination, treatment for physical injuries, and tests for STIs.

Sexual assault is a crime and should be reported to law enforcement. Police can arrest the person who committed the assault if they know what occurred and can collect evidence. As a result, a person who experiences sexual assault should not change clothes or shower before going to the police station or hospital. Professionals can gather evidence from clothes and hair.

Many people who experienced sexual assault find it helpful to receive counseling. Some people find support by talking to others who have been through this trauma. A school nurse, doctor, or local crisis center can provide information about counselors and local support groups. People might also find it useful to talk to other adults they trust. Parents or guardians, a family physician, community leaders, and teachers are examples.

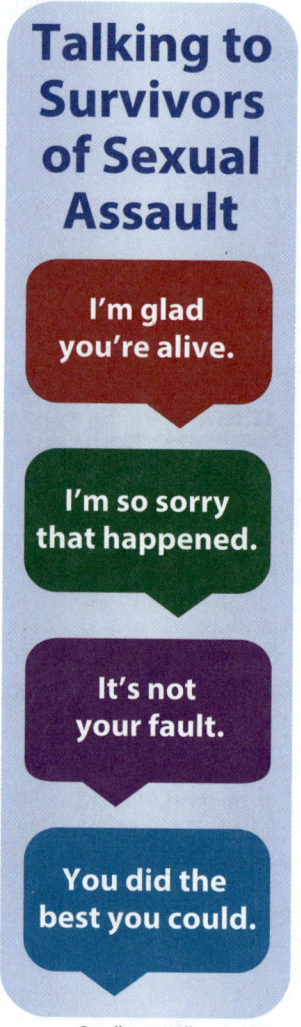

Goodheart-Willcox Publisher

Figure 9.2.8
Sometimes, it can be hard to know what to say to a survivor of sexual assault. The messages in this illustration can be helpful and can convey that you care.

Supporting Survivors of Sexual Assault

If you know a person who has experienced sexual assault, understand that the person may or may not want to talk about the attack. Follow the person's lead and do not ask too many questions. Try to be a good listener. Do not judge the person's behavior or blame the person for what happened (**Figure 9.2.8**). Encourage the person to seek professional help or talk to a parent or other trusted adult. Remember, the person who experienced sexual assault is never to blame.

9.2–5 Reading Checkpoint

1. What is the best way to prevent sexual assault? Explain.
2. If sexual assault occurs, what should a person do immediately after the event?

Lesson 9.2 Review and Assessment

Reading Summary

9.2–1 Sexual violence is sexual behavior that occurs without legal consent. Legal consent is a direct, verbal, and freely given agreement given by someone older than the age of consent.

9.2–2 Sexual harassment is verbal or nonverbal sexual attention that occurs without legal consent.

9.2–3 When someone is sexually harassed, people can be upstanders. They can get the person away, get adults to help, or record what happened.

9.2–4 Sexual assault is threatening or forcing someone into sexual activity. It is illegal and a crime. Sexual assault can cause physical injuries and lead to anxiety and depression.

9.2–5 Sexual assault is never the fault of the survivor. To prevent sexual assault, understand and respect consent and avoid risky settings. After a sexual assault, call 911 and seek medical help. People can listen to and support survivors.

Critical Thinking

1. **Assess.** Why might it be difficult for a young person to refuse an unwanted kiss, touch, or other form of sexual activity in a relationship? Defend your answer.
2. **Analyze.** What populations, communities, or groups of individuals may have limited access to services that support people who have experienced sexual assault? What could be done to increase their access to services?

Develop Your Skills

1. **Practice Health-Enhancing Behaviors.** For this activity, imagine that in class, a student beside you starts to make sexual comments about you. The comments make you feel uncomfortable. Reflect on how you would respond to protect your health and safety. Then, share your answers with a partner and discuss other ways to respond. After sharing your responses with your classmate, role-play what you could do in these situations.
2. **Communicate with Others.** With a partner, practice responding to the following statements. If you would feel unsafe responding in the situation, describe what you would do instead.
   - **Scenario 1:** You have been asked out several times by an individual. You have politely declined each time. During lunch, the individual comes up to you and states, "Have you changed your mind yet? I want to go out with you."
   - **Scenario 2:** While walking through the hall, another student comes up behind you and feels your backside, stating, "I like the way it looks in your jeans."
   - **Scenario 3:** You briefly dated another student at your school but broke up after two weeks. While hanging out with friends at lunch, a classmate tells you that the person you dated is spreading rumors about what happened sexually in your relationship.
3. **Access Information.** Various resources are available to help people who experience sexual assault. Research valid sources to learn more about options to help those who experience sexual assault. Research three categories: getting help from home, getting help at school, and getting help in the community. For each category, list resources available, benefits of the resource, location of the resource or service, the cost (if applicable), and other relevant information. Create a graphic organizer or mind map to organize and display your information.

Lesson 9.3: Abuse and Neglect

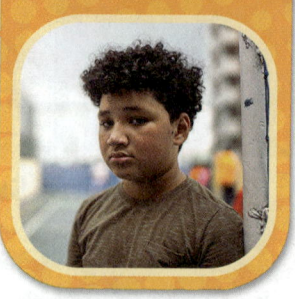

Key Terms

abuse violent behaviors that cause physical, emotional, sexual, or financial harm to another person

physical abuse behaviors that cause physical harm to a person

emotional abuse attitudes or controlling behaviors that harm mental health

sexual abuse sexual activity to which one person does not or cannot legally consent

financial abuse use of money to show power in a relationship and make others act in certain ways

intimate partner violence abuse that involves two people who are or were in a romantic relationship

child abuse any intentional act by an adult that causes harm or threatens to cause harm to a child

neglect type of child abuse in which a child's basic physical, emotional, medical, or educational needs are not met by parents or guardians

sibling abuse violent behaviors that one sibling inflicts on another sibling

elder abuse behaviors or neglect that cause harm to someone 60 years of age or older

Learning Outcomes

Look for the skills icon  to practice health skills.
After studying this lesson, you will be able to

- 9.3–1 **Identify** the types of abuse and the patterns of power and control in abuse.
- 9.3–2 **Explain** what intimate partner violence is.
- 9.3–3 **Summarize** the effects of child abuse.
- 9.3–4 **List** forms of sibling abuse and elder abuse.
- 9.3–5 **Identify** strategies for preventing and responding to abuse.

Essential Question

What are different types of abuse, and how can abuse be prevented?

Reading and Notetaking Activity

As you read the lesson, assign a category to each section based on the different topics covered in the lesson. Write the topic in each section. Fill the organizer with your notes on different types of abuse and neglect.

Topic: Sibling Abuse	Topic:
Notes: Sibling abuse is not the same as sibling conflict or rivalry.	Notes:
Topic:	**Topic:**
Notes:	Notes:
Topic:	**Topic:**
Notes:	Notes:

Goodheart-Willcox Publisher

Lesson image:
FG Trade/iStock/Getty Images Plus
via Getty Images

Introduction

Healthy relationships do not have violent behavior or abuse. For example, Sofia's friend Tad is always fighting with his mother. During disagreements, his mother sometimes calls him names. She has even shoved him out of the house before.

Sofia is unsure of how to help her friend. Tad thinks his mother's behavior is normal. Sofia knows, however, that all types of abuse are wrong.

9.3-1 Types of Abuse

Abuse is the violent mistreatment of a person. For example, hitting someone when you are angry is abuse. Shaking a sibling is also abuse. Abuse is not always physical. People can use words, attitudes, and behaviors to abuse another person (Figure 9.3.1). The following are types of abuse:

- **Physical abuse** involves actions that cause physical harm to another person. Physical abuse may involve hitting, kicking, choking, slapping, biting, shaking, or burning someone.
- **Emotional abuse** involves attitudes or behaviors that harm a person's mental and emotional health. This is also called *mental*, *verbal*, or *psychological abuse*. It includes making threats, calling someone names, delivering insults, making fun of someone's identity, withholding love, and isolating a person.
- **Sexual abuse** involves sexual activity to which one person does not or cannot legally consent. Sexual abuse can include physical behaviors such as unwanted sexual activity. Sexual abuse can also involve other activities, such as sexual harassment *flashing* (exposing one's self), sending someone a nude picture, or asking someone to send you a nude picture.

> **Essential Idea**
> Abuse can take many different forms, including physical, emotional, sexual, and financial.

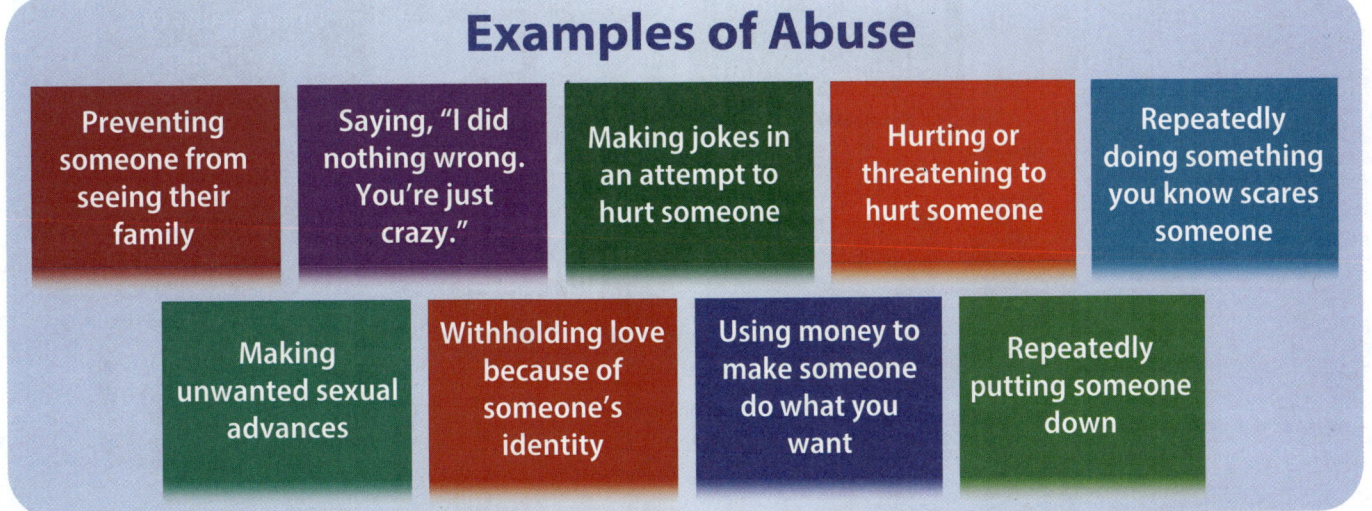

Figure 9.3.1 Many different actions can be abuse. These all involve violent, consistent mistreatment of another person.

- **Financial abuse** is the use of money to show power in a relationship. It could include stealing or giving gifts or money and expecting something in return. Financial abuse may also involve withholding money to meet basic needs.

Abuse can occur in families. It can also occur between friends, among classmates, or between dating partners. In all of these settings, abuse has serious physical and emotional consequences. It can sometimes be a crime (**Figure 9.3.2**).

Abusive behavior aims to take power or control over the person being abused. Abuse can take many forms (**Figure 9.3.3**).

Abuse sometimes involves four stages. This is called the *cycle of abuse*. These stages include tension building, incident, reconciliation, and calm.

In *tension building*, one person grows angry. It feels like the other person is "walking on eggshells." Then the *incident*, or any type of abuse, occurs. During *reconciliation*, the person who committed the abuse may apologize, blame the person being abused, or deny that the abuse happened. In the *calm* stage, the person who committed the abuse acts like it never happened. They may give gifts to the person being abused. It may seem like the abuse is over, until tension builds again.

Not all abuse follows this cycle. However, these stages can help people recognize abusive behavior. Abuse is a pattern of power and control. The abuse does not stop unless the pattern is broken.

Signs of Abuse

Physical Signs
- Bruises, black eyes, welts, burns, cuts, broken bones

Social and Emotional Signs
- Anxiety, extreme upset
- Nervousness and fear around certain people
- Changes in behavior
- Withdrawal from relationships and social activities
- Concern with being alone at night
- Nightmares and bedwetting

Goodheart-Willcox Publisher

Figure 9.3.2 Abuse is a crime. It can have serious physical, social, and emotional consequences.

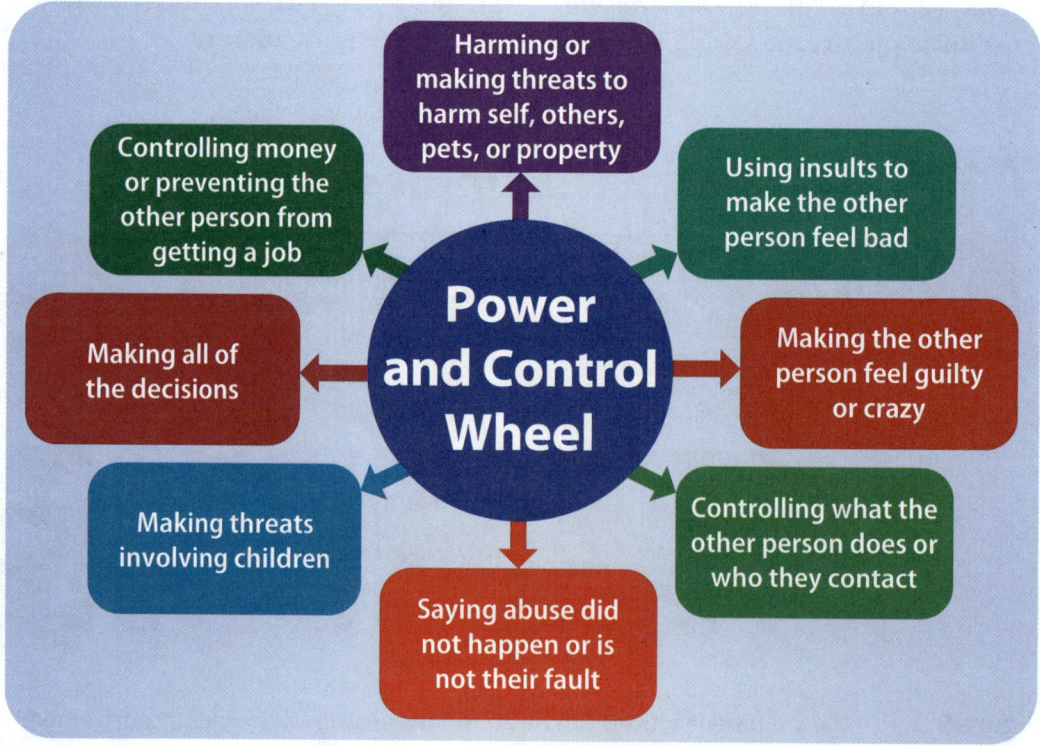

Figure 9.3.3 The power and control wheel describes common forms of abuse.

Goodheart-Willcox Publisher

Often, people try to make those they abuse feel responsible for the abuse. This is *never* the case. The person committing the abuse is *always* responsible for the abuse. Some examples of abuse are intimate partner violence, child abuse, sibling abuse, and elder abuse. Peer abuse and bullying or cyberbullying are also examples of abuse.

9.3-1 Reading Checkpoint

1. Describe what abuse is. Include the different forms of abuse in your response.
2. Explain how power and control factor into abuse.

9.3-2 Intimate Partner Violence

Intimate partner violence is abuse between two people who are or were married, dating, or in a romantic relationship. Intimate partner violence is also called *domestic violence*, *spousal violence*, or *dating violence*. Intimate partner violence occurs when one or both partners try to dominate or control the other. This involves physical, emotional, sexual, or financial abuse. It can occur in person or online.

Certain signs indicate abuse in a relationship (**Figure 9.3.4**). These can include physical injuries, such as bruises or broken bones. These signs may also include depression, anxiety, fear, and shame.

People who experience intimate partner violence may feel socially isolated and alone. This may be partly because they do not want to tell anyone.

> **Essential Idea**
> Intimate partner violence is abuse between two people who are or were married, dating, or in a romantic relationship.

Signs of Intimate Partner Violence

It could be intimate partner violence if your partner...

- gets upset when you spend time with others
- does not take responsibility for actions
- blames you or uses emotions to manipulate you
- gets angry easily, gets violent, or tries to scare you during conflicts
- puts you down and does not listen to your concerns
- pressures you or does not respect your boundaries

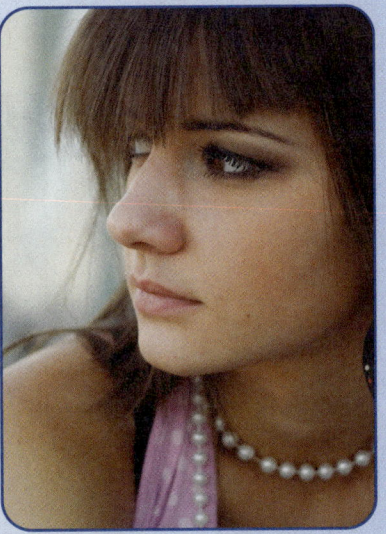

Ardelean Andreea/Shutterstock.com

Figure 9.3.4 Intimate partner violence often starts with emotional abuse. It may turn to physical abuse. It can occur in dating relationships and in marriages.

Lesson Abuse and Neglect

Intimate partner violence can also negatively affect other people. Children who see violence can develop anxiety, depression, or suicidal thoughts. They can also act out violently themselves.

Healthy relationships do not include abuse and violence. There is never a good reason for violent behavior. You should leave a relationship if a partner behaves violently. Get out the *very first time* violence occurs. Staying in a relationship with a partner who makes you feel uncomfortable or scared can be dangerous. Intimate partner violence is also illegal. It should always be reported.

9.3–2 Reading Checkpoint

1. What is intimate partner abuse? Include the signs of this abuse in your response.
2. What should a person do if their partner behaves violently?

9.3-3 Child Abuse

Essential Idea
Child abuse and neglect is an intentional act by an adult that causes harm or threatens to cause harm to a child.

Each year in the United States, nearly 700,000 children are abused or neglected. Some children die from abuse or neglect each year. **Child abuse** is any intentional act by an adult that causes harm or threatens to cause harm to a child.

Types of Child Neglect and Abuse

Child abuse can take many forms. For example, it can mean withholding love or being emotionally distant. It can also include ignoring a child.

Child sexual abuse is when an adult engages a child in any sexual activity. It may involve the use of pressure, force, or deception. Child sexual abuse can include kissing, touching, having the child view sexual images, or looking at the child sexually (Figure 9.3.5). Any adult who engages in sexual activity with a child can be charged with a crime.

Figure 9.3.5 Young people under a certain age cannot legally consent to sexual activities.

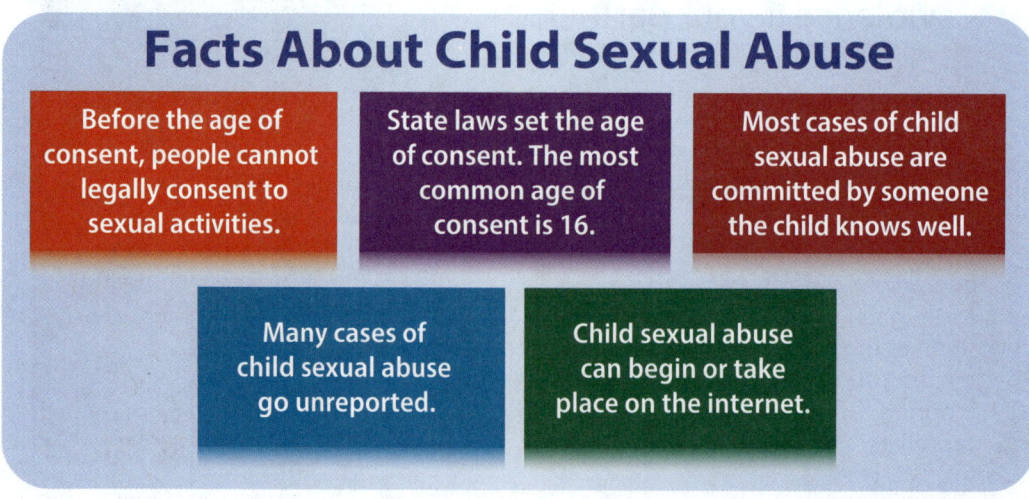

Facts About Child Sexual Abuse

- Before the age of consent, people cannot legally consent to sexual activities.
- State laws set the age of consent. The most common age of consent is 16.
- Most cases of child sexual abuse are committed by someone the child knows well.
- Many cases of child sexual abuse go unreported.
- Child sexual abuse can begin or take place on the internet.

Goodheart-Willcox Publisher

Another type of child abuse is neglect. **Neglect** is when an adult fails to meet a child's basic physical, emotional, medical, or educational needs. Neglect also includes failing to protect a child from harm. For example, the child may not be well supervised. A child may have an unsafe living situation. A child may not have enough food or warm clothes (**Figure 9.3.6**).

Effects of Child Neglect and Abuse

A child's sense of well-being comes from their family and caregivers. Children need love, support, and respect from those around them. Abuse and neglect harm children's sense of well-being. This can have serious consequences on children's health.

Child abuse or neglect can have physical consequences. These can include the following:

- severe bruises
- broken bones
- burns
- brain damage
- delayed development
- malnutrition

Children who are abused are also more likely to develop health conditions and diseases. They have an increased risk of abusing tobacco, alcohol, and drugs.

Children who are abused or neglected also have a greater risk of mental health conditions. These include the following:

- depression
- anxiety
- eating disorders
- post-traumatic stress disorder (PTSD)

Ongoing abuse may cause children to develop learning, attention, and memory issues. This can lead to difficulty in school.

Risk Factors for Child Abuse and Neglect

- Expensive or unavailable healthcare
- Unplanned pregnancy
- Teen pregnancy
- Emotional immaturity
- Difficult family relationships
- Lack of knowledge about parenting and child development
- Many children in the home or very young children
- Use of physical punishment for discipline
- Premature birth or low birthweight
- Dislike of child
- Disobedience and arguing
- Frequent crying
- History of early aggressive behavior
- Exposure to violence, abuse, and conflict in the family
- Use of tobacco, alcohol, or drugs
- Discrimination and bias
- Low level of family eduction and income
- High crime and unemployment rates

Goodheart-Willcox Publisher

Figure 9.3.6 Certain risk factors increase the risk for child abuse and neglect.

Child abuse or neglect can make it harder for a person to build and maintain healthy relationships. People who are abused may have trouble forming healthy relationships as adults.

Pay attention to the signs of child abuse and neglect. This can help you identify if this violent behavior is occurring (Figure 9.3.7).

Figure 9.3.7 Some people who are abused blame themselves, but abuse is always the fault of the person committing the abuse. The person being abused is never responsible for abuse.

Difficulty sleeping is a sign of which type of abuse?

Signs of Child Abuse and Neglect

Types of Abuse	Signs
Physical abuse	• Injuries, such as broken bones or severe bruises • Many injuries on different parts of he body • Several injuries that occurred at different times
Sexual abuse	• Bruises in the pelvic area • Difficulty or pain when walking or sitting • Torn clothing
Emotional abuse	• Withdrawn attitude and unwillingness to talk to others • Anxiety or worry • Difficulty sleeping • Aggressive or inappropriate behavior
Neglect	• Underweight • Poor physical development • Lack of cleanliness

Goodheart-Willcox Publisher

9.3-3 Reading Checkpoint

1. Describe the different forms of child abuse and include how these forms can affect the child's health and well-being.
2. How can middle school students benefit from learning the signs of child abuse?

Essential Idea

Sibling abuse is the physical, emotional, or sexual mistreatment of one sibling by another. Elder abuse is the physical, emotional, sexual, or financial abuse or neglect of an older adult.

9.3-4 Sibling and Elder Abuse

People with siblings and older adults are two groups who can experience specific forms of abuse.

Sibling Abuse

Sibling abuse is the violent mistreatment of one sibling by another. Sibling abuse can be physical, emotional, or sexual. It has serious health consequences. Sibling abuse is a common type of family abuse. It often occurs in families where other unhealthy relationships exist.

72 Module Violence

CASE STUDY

Aarav and Rajesh: Boys Will Be Boys

Aarav is 12 years old. He is scared of his older brother Rajesh. Rajesh always taunts Aarav about his weight. He calls him "fatty" or "doughboy." Sometimes he pinches the fat around his waist or on his arms.

Aarav became very upset one day. He told his dad about Rajesh's mean comments and actions. His father told Rajesh to stop teasing his brother. That did not work, though. Rajesh's teasing only got worse.

Often, Aarav's parents work late. This means that Rajesh is in charge at home. Rajesh yells at Aarav to do all the chores. If Aarav resists, Rajesh will hit, kick, and push him. Aarav tries to stay out of his brother's way. Rajesh tells Aarav that he will hurt him more if he tells anyone about their fights. A few times, Aarav has had to hide the scrapes and bruises. He does not want his parents or people at school to ask about them.

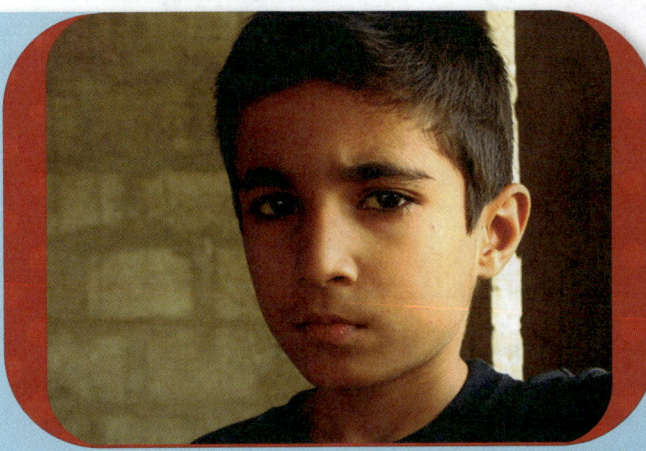

iStock.com/danishkhan

 Practice Your Skills — **Advocate for Health**

Write a short health-enhancing message answering the following questions:
- What challenge is Aarav facing?
- Does Aarav need help with this situation? Why or why not?
- Who would be helpful adults in this situation? What would be the best way to get help from them?
- When, where, and how would you suggest Aarav connect with these helpful adults?

Some conflict or rivalry is normal between siblings. Abuse, however, is not normal. Unlike rivalry, abuse is part of an ongoing pattern. Sibling abuse is typically one-sided. It aims to dominate the person being abused.

Elder Abuse

Elder abuse is the abuse of an older adult. It can occur in older adults' homes, nursing homes, or other living situations. Typically, family members or

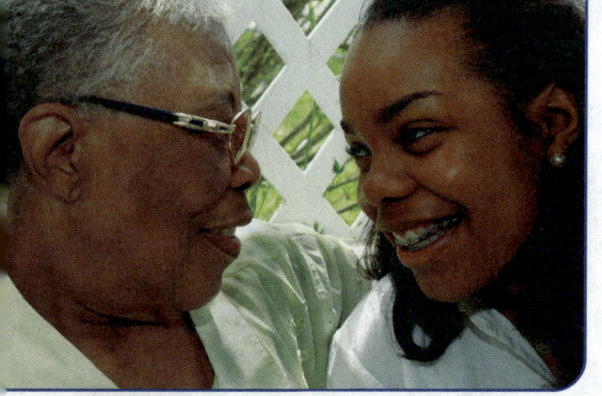

paid caregivers commit elder abuse. Elder abuse can include the following:
- physical abuse, including inappropriate use of medications or restraints
- emotional abuse, including ignoring calls for help or saying cruel words
- sexual abuse
- financial abuse, including theft of money or property
- neglect, including failure to provide food, water, medications, and basic hygiene

iStock.com/nano

Figure 9.3.8 Some older adults rely on their families or caregivers for help with daily needs. They need loved ones to protect them from harm. If this care is not provided, older adults can be severely hurt by abuse or neglect.

Older adults who are abused or neglected often feel helpless, lonely, and distressed. They also tend to die earlier than older adults who have not been abused (**Figure 9.3.8**).

9.3-4 Reading Checkpoint

1. How is sibling abuse different than sibling rivalry?
2. What are examples of elder abuse?
3. What is the impact of elder abuse on the individual who is abused?

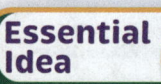

Essential Idea

To prevent abuse from happening or continuing, promote health for yourself and others, leave an abusive situation, and report abuse.

9.3-5 Preventing and Responding to Abuse

Many communities take steps to prevent abuse. Organizations and government agencies may provide programs or online resources to educate people about abuse. You can help prevent abuse using the following strategies.

Promote Health

One way to help prevent abuse is to promote health for yourself, your family, and your community. You can promote health in the following ways:
- People who experience abuse sometimes abuse others. If you have been abused, talk to a mental health professional.
- Develop communication and conflict resolution skills.
- Build and maintain healthy relationships.
- Recognize situations that increase the risk of abuse. This includes the use of drugs and alcohol.
- Find ways to value diversity. Show respect for other people and their perspectives.
- Seek treatment for mental health conditions and illnesses.

74 Module Violence

Responding to Abuse

Steps for responding to abuse include the following:

1. **Recognize the abusive situation.** Do not make excuses. There is never a good reason for abuse. Talking with a parent or other trusted adult can help you identify abuse.
2. **Remember that abuse may seem to stop.** This does not mean the abuse is over or is not real. Even if the person acting abusively is being nice, the abuse still needs to be addressed.
3. **Do not try to change the person who is being abusive.** That person needs professional help.
4. **Leave or help someone leave an abusive relationship or situation.** Sometimes it may seem unsafe to leave. Talk with a parent or other trusted adult or call a hotline about how to leave. Try to leave when it is safe. Crisis shelters can provide safety.
5. **Block the person who is being abusive from contacting you.** You may need to do this if you need to do more than physically leave an abusive situation.

Report Abuse

Recognizing abuse and neglect is the first step to stopping it. Some laws require children and teens to learn about signs of abuse.

For example, Erin's Law requires that children and teens be taught about body safety to recognize sexual abuse and to speak up if they are being abused.

Anyone who thinks a person is being abused should report this to an authority. This could be a police officer, teacher, nurse, or doctor. It could also be a parent, guardian, or other trusted adult. Several hotlines can also help people experiencing abuse (**Figure 9.3.9**).

Some jobs require people to report abuse. People in these jobs are called *mandated reporters*. They include the following:

- teachers and other school personnel
- social workers and child welfare workers
- healthcare professionals

A state organization, such as a child welfare agency or law enforcement, will talk with anyone who may have information about abuse. If they find abuse occurred, they may make an arrest.

Children who are abused may be placed in foster care. *Foster care* is an arrangement in which adults agree to care for children who are not legally theirs.

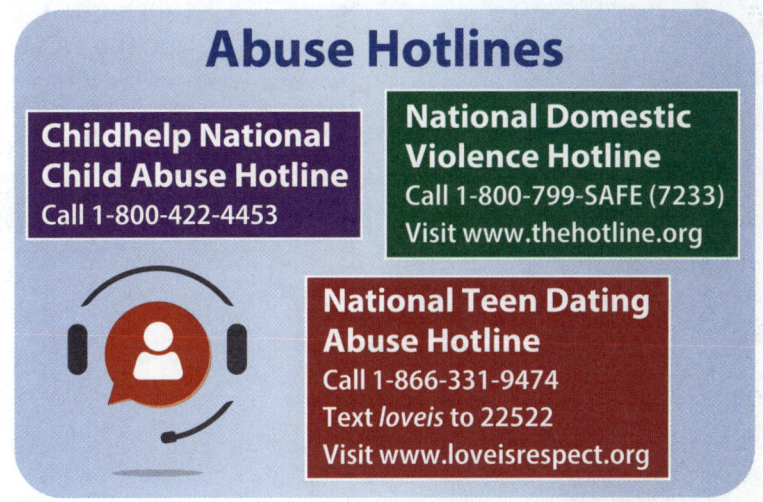

vladwel/Shutterstock.com

Figure 9.3.9 Abuse hotlines can help people report abuse. They can also help people leave abusive situations.

People who commit abuse may be required to receive treatment. They may be charged with a crime and sent to prison.

Get Help and Treatment

Someone who has been abused should seek medical treatment for any injuries caused by abuse. For example, a person could go to a hospital or urgent care center. A crisis shelter can provide safety after a person leaves an abusive situation.

Seeking professional help after escaping abuse is important. Mental health therapy sessions provide a safe space to share feelings, thoughts, and fears. This process can help people have healthier relationships. Therapists can help people with the following:

- sharing feelings, thoughts, and fears
- working through experiences
- managing bad memories
- coping with anxiety, anger, and fear

If you or someone you know has been abused, talk to a trusted adult. This could be a parent, guardian, teacher, school counselor, or nurse. That adult can help you find help from a trained professional.

People who commit abuse or neglect also need professional help. Parents or guardians who abuse may need education on parenting techniques. People who commit sexual abuse may need training to increase empathy and self-control.

9.3–5 Reading Checkpoint

1. How can a person prevent abuse? Provide a detailed response with examples.
2. What should a person do if they think someone is being abused?
3. What are help and treatment options for a person who has experienced abuse?

Lesson 9.3 Review and Assessment

Reading Summary

9.3–1 The consistent, violent mistreatment of a person is abuse. Abuse can be physical, emotional, sexual, or financial. Abuse aims to take power or control over the person being abused.

9.3–2 Intimate partner violence is abuse that involves two people who are or were in a romantic relationship.

9.3–3 Child abuse is an intentional act that causes harm or threatens to cause harm to a child. Neglect is when an adult fails to meet a child's basic needs.

9.3–4 Sibling abuse is the mistreatment of one sibling by another. This can be physical, emotional, or sexual. Older adults who are mistreated experience elder abuse.

9.3–5 To prevent abuse, promote health for yourself and others. If abuse happens, leave the abusive situation and report the abuse.

Critical Thinking

1. **Evaluate.** Why do you think experiencing abuse or neglect makes a person more likely to abuse or neglect others? How can abuse be a cycle over generations?
2. **Determine.** Often, people remain silent about difficult situations that involve abuse or neglect. How can silence allow the abuse or neglect to keep happening?

Develop Your Skills

1. **Communicate with Others.** Although it is never fun, talking about abuse and neglect can make it easier for people to reach out for help. With a partner, create a scenario where you have concerns that someone is being abused or neglected. Together, talk about what you could do to help this person.
2. **Access Information.** Identify five agencies in your local and national community that assist people affected by abusive or neglectful behavior. These can be resources for people who experience abuse or neglect, people who commit abuse or neglect, or family members of those impacted by abuse or neglect. Create a resource list with each agency's name, contact information, mission statement, and service or services provided.
3. **Make Decisions.** Imagine that you suspect a close friend is being abused by an adult that they trust and spend a significant amount of time with. Using a decision-making model, explore your options for responding to this information and make a decision about what to do. Be prepared to share your options, your final decision, and an explanation of why you made that decision.

Lesson 9.4

Violence in the Community

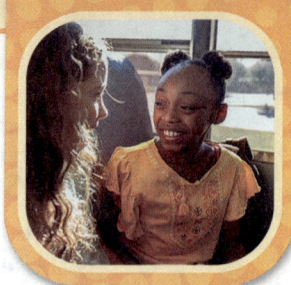

Key Terms

school violence violent behavior that occurs at any school-related event

gangs groups of people who carry out violent and illegal acts

human trafficking form of modern slavery which involves people forcing or pressuring someone to perform a job or service

hate crimes threats or violence against someone based on their race, ethnic origin, disability, sex, or religion

homicide crime of killing another person

terrorism use of violence and threats to frighten and control people to promote a political or religious view

Learning Outcomes

Look for the skills icon  to practice health skills.
After studying this lesson, you will be able to

9.4–1 **Explain** what school violence is and how to prevent it.
9.4–2 **Describe** the reasons for and consequences of joining gangs.
9.4–3 **List** ways to protect yourself from human trafficking.
9.4–4 **Describe** how to prevent hate crimes.
9.4–5 **Identify** ways to prevent homicide and terrorism.
9.4–6 **Explain** how to prevent violence.

Essential Question

What forms can violence take in your community and how can you prevent violence?

Reading and Notetaking Activity

Review the learning outcomes and key terms for the lesson. Then, create a KWL chart. Before reading this lesson, write what you know and what you want to know about to these types of violence and violence prevention strategies. After studying the lesson, write what you have learned.

K: What I Know
Violent behavior and threats should be reported to a trusted adult.

W: What I Want to Know
What are other ways to prevent or reduce violence?

L: What I Have Learned
Practicing conflict-resolution skills, building healthy relationships, and practicing safety at home are all ways to help prevent violence.

Goodheart-Willcox Publisher

Lesson image:
SDI Productions/E+ via Getty Images

Introduction

Lately, Ravi has been watching the news with his parents. As he learns more about the world, he feels more afraid. He worries violence will impact his community.

Stories about gang violence and terrorism make Ravi afraid. He worries about going to public events. Ravi wants to know how to avoid and prevent violence.

Violence can occur anywhere, even in places where people should feel safe. In this lesson, you will learn about different types of violent behavior. You will also learn ways to respond to and prevent violence.

9.4-1 School Violence

School violence is violent behavior that occurs at any school-related event. This includes more than just violence during school (Figure 9.4.1). School violence can include bullying and cyberbullying. It also includes fighting and the use of weapons.

All students should feel safe at school. School violence, however, puts many students in danger. For example, a fight might seem like it only affects two students, but if a fight gets out of control, other students can get hurt. Especially if a student brings a weapon to school, other students can be hurt or even die. Emotionally, students who see violence can feel depressed, anxious, and fearful.

Violence in schools can have serious consequences. It can lead to detention, suspension, or expulsion. It can also lead to an arrest.

Many schools have violence-prevention programs which work to prevent and reduce violence. Violence-prevention programs use the following strategies:

- Select positive, responsible student leaders. These leaders act appropriately. They are not afraid to speak out against violence.
- Develop team-building activities to strengthen bonds among students.

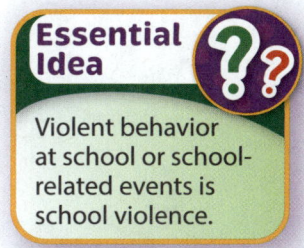

Essential Idea

Violent behavior at school or school-related events is school violence.

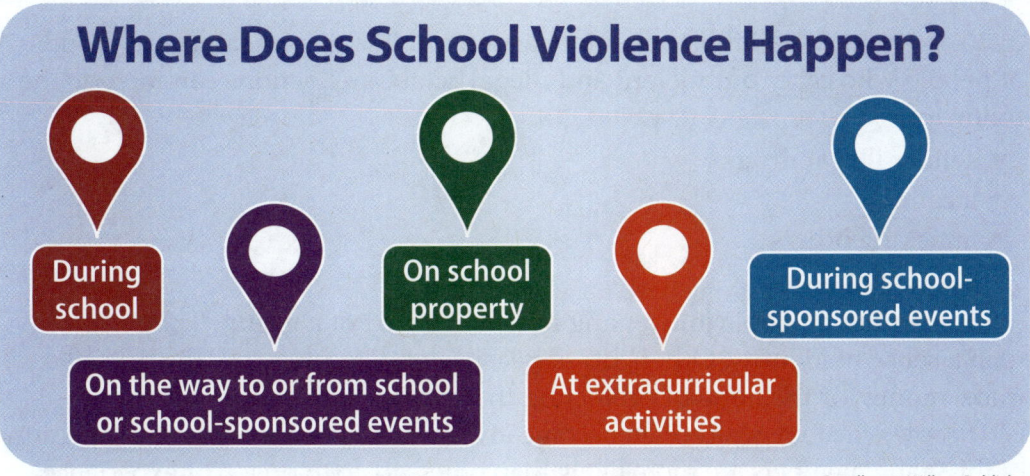

Figure 9.4.1 School violence can happen at school. It can also occur in other locations.

Is violence on the school bus considered school violence? Why or why not?

Goodheart-Willcox Publisher

TELL SOMEONE if you
- see a weapon
- witness or hear about any violent act
- hear or see one student threaten another
- see someone suspicious in or near the school
- hear about or see any plans to commit violence

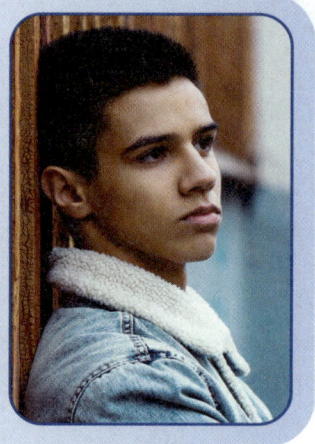

Malivan_Iuliia/Shutterstock.com

Figure 9.4.2 Immediately alert adults to violent behaviors. They can prevent or stop dangerous situations. Some schools offer anonymous ways of reporting.

- Treat violent behavior seriously. Any violence results in consequences.
- Have a buddy system where older students look out for younger students.
- Encourage students to immediately report any violent acts they observe (**Figure 9.4.2**).
- Enforce rules about locking school doors.
- Ensure a weapon-free student population. Communicate rules about weapons. Search students' belongings as necessary.
- Offer peer mediation programs. This can prevent conflicts from escalating.

Students play an important role in preventing violence. Following the rules of violence prevention programs is the only way for programs to be effective in reducing and preventing violence. For example, when students follow rules about locking school doors, the school can keep dangerous people out of the building.

9.4-1 Reading Checkpoint

1. How does school violence affect students?
2. Review the strategies of a successful school violence prevention program. Which of these strategies is your school currently doing or could do better to prevent violence?

9.4-2 Gang Violence

Essential Idea
Groups of people who commit violent and illegal acts are called *gangs*.

Gang violence is violent behavior carried out in a gang. **Gangs** are groups of people who carry out violent and illegal acts. Gang actions can include the following:
- selling illegal drugs
- stealing
- attacking others
- damaging property

Some young people join a gang to feel like part of a group. They want to gain a sense of identity. Others do so because of peer pressure, the desire to make money, or the hope of protecting themselves and their families.

People who join gangs often become involved in violence and crimes. Because of this, gang members are more likely than others to go to prison or experience violence. They may drop out of school, be unable to find a job, or develop an addiction to drugs. Committing a crime can severely impact a person's future. Many gang members also lose their lives to violence.

Communities often have resources that help reduce gang violence. For example, officials may try to limit the size and reach of gangs. To be successful, city workers and police officers must be deeply involved in the community and build trust. **Figure 9.4.3** lists some strategies you can use for avoiding gang violence.

Figure 9.4.3 Many communities try to help young people avoid gang violence. They can help you use these strategies.

What can you do if you feel pressured to join a gang?

9.4-2 Reading Checkpoint

1. Why might a young person join a gang?
2. What are communities doing to reduce gang violence?

9.4-3 Human Trafficking

Human trafficking is a form of modern slavery. It involves forcing or pressuring someone to perform a job or service. Human trafficking is a crime.

There are different types of trafficking. In *labor trafficking*, employers use threats to force people to work. In *sex trafficking*, people are forced to engage in sexual activity. This is called *sexual exploitation*.

In human trafficking, violence, drugs, and coercion are used to make people do something. People who traffic others are often in a position of power over the person being trafficked. This power imbalance can be based on the following:

- age
- gender
- income
- immigration status
- race

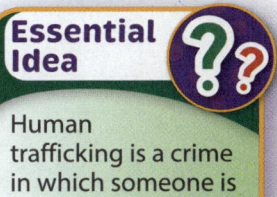

Essential Idea

Human trafficking is a crime in which someone is forced or pressured into performing a job or service.

Sometimes, trafficking begins with kidnapping. More often, people trick others with promises. For example, a person may reach out to young people on social media and ask to meet. Human trafficking can also begin in a relationship. One person may force their partner to work or engage in sexual activity.

Human trafficking has serious consequences. People who are trafficked may experience fatigue, pain, injuries, infections, and pregnancy. They may develop mental health conditions, such as depression, anxiety, substance use disorders, or PTSD. Often, people who are trafficked do not have or are separated from healthy, supportive relationships.

Taking precautions can help you avoid human trafficking. These can include the following:

- Lock the doors and windows at home.
- Do not go anywhere with someone you do not know well.
- Do not meet someone you know online in person without supervision.
- Do not give out your personal information.
- Avoid using substances such as drugs and alcohol.

Sometimes the person who traffics others gives gifts or money. They may make promises. These behaviors may be *grooming*, which means building a relationship in order to take advantage of someone (especially a young person). Be cautious if someone offers you a job that seems too good to be true. Reach out to a parent, guardian, or other trusted adult.

Leave a relationship if you feel unsafe, or if the other person has more power. Talk to a parent, guardian, or other trusted adult for help.

Know the signs of human trafficking. This can help you identify if you or others are being groomed or trafficked. Report any suspected cases of human trafficking (Figure 9.4.4).

Figure 9.4.4 People who are trafficked need help. Learn the signs of human trafficking. Alert the authorities to any suspected cases in your community.

Signs of Human Trafficking

- Unexplained, regular school absences
- Running away from home
- Regular travel
- Bruises or other physical injuries
- Lack of control over schedule
- Hunger
- Sudden changes in behavior or hygiene
- Dodging questions or lying
- Older romantic partner
- Lack of concentration
- Anxiety, anger, and depression

If you suspect human trafficking:
- **talk** to a parent or other trusted adult
- **visit** humantraffickinghotline.org/chat
- **call** the National Human Trafficking Hotline (1-888-373-7888)
- **text** HELP to BeFree (233733)

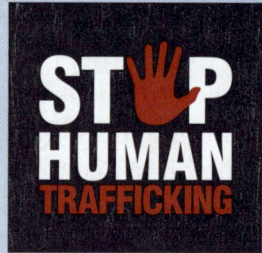

ria_airborne/Shutterstock.com

9.4–3 Reading Checkpoint

1. What are strategies to prevent human trafficking?
2. What should you do if you suspect human trafficking?

9.4-4 Hate Crimes

Hate crimes are threats or violence against someone based on their race, ethnic origin, disability, sex, or religion. People who commit hate crimes see the person they attack as a symbol of a larger group. Because of this, hate crimes can hurt entire communities.

Hate crimes include the following:
- physical attacks
- emotional attacks
- damaging property
- making threats

People who experience a hate crime can experience a physical injury or loss of property. They may also experience mental health conditions. Physical injuries and mental health conditions may require medical treatment.

Committing a hate crime can lead to school consequences, such as suspension or expulsion. Committing a hate crime can also result in legal consequences since most states have laws against hate crimes.

Hate crimes are motivated by prejudice and bias. Instead, celebrate differences. Encourage others to do the same. Appreciating diversity can help reduce hate crimes.

> **Essential Idea**
>
> Violence or threats of violence against someone because of their race, ethnic origin, disability, sex, or religion is a hate crime.

9.4-4 Reading Checkpoint

1. What are hate crimes?
2. What are the consequences of experiencing a hate crime? of committing a hate crime?

9.4-5 Homicide and Terrorism

Killing someone is a very serious crime called a **homicide**. Homicides occur through physical injury. For example, attacking another student can lead to homicide. So can using a weapon at school. Homicides lead to serious, lasting consequences.

Homicide ends another person's life. It devastates families, friends, and communities. Homicide leads to serious criminal charges. Young people who commit homicide may spend the rest of their life in prison.

The best way to prevent homicide is to report violent behavior to trusted adults. Take threats of homicide seriously. Tell a parent, guardian, school official, teacher, or other adult. Immediately report any weapons or violent situations you see at school or in your community. This can allow an adult to intervene to prevent a homicide. Avoiding weapons can reduce harm caused by them.

Terrorism is the use of violence and threats to frighten and control people. It may involve killing or injuring people to promote a political

> **Essential Idea**
>
> Killing someone is called a *homicide*, and it is a very serious crime. Terrorism uses violence and threats to frighten and control people.

or religious view. Most terrorism is caused by violent extremism. *Violent extremism* involves using violence to promote an idea. For example, someone might hurt people who practice a certain religion.

Terrorism creates fear in communities. It does not validate a person's viewpoint. Terrorism is a serious crime. You can help prevent terrorism by reporting any suspicious activity (**Figure 9.4.5**). If you report suspicious activity, you should describe what you saw. Explain when and where you saw it and why it is suspicious.

Another way to prevent terrorism is to celebrate differences between people. Encourage others to celebrate diversity too. This can help reduce violent extremism.

Figure 9.4.5 Certain activities may be signs of terrorism. Report any suspicious activity to the police.

What Is Suspicious Activity?

Unusual objects or situations
- An unfamiliar car parked in a strange location
- An unattended bag or backpack in a public place
- A person lingering outside a school

Requesting information
- A person who wants to know how to get into your school
- A person who wants to know your club's exact schedule and location

Observation
- A person who sits in a car outside your school every day
- A person measuring and taking pictures of a community facility

Goodheart-Willcox Publisher

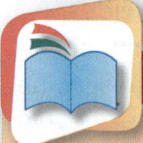

9.4–5 Reading Checkpoint

1. How can homicide be prevented?
2. What is terrorism?
3. What makes an activity suspicious? What should you do if you see suspicious activity?

9.4-6 Responding to and Preventing Violence

Violence can have serious physical and emotional effects. This includes physical injuries and feelings of helplessness.

Know how to respond to violence. Your actions can affect your well-being and the well-being of others. The following strategies can help you respond to violent behavior:

- If someone uses or threatens violence, tell a trusted adult. This could be a parent, guardian, school official, or the police.
- Get out of violent relationships. There is no excuse for violence.
- Get medical help for physical injuries. Get professional help to manage the emotional impact of violence.

Everyone in a community, including you, can help reduce and prevent violence. You can recognize the signs of violence and reduce risk factors. Behaving in a nonviolent manner is another way you can reduce violence (**Figure 9.4.6**).

The following strategies can help you prevent and reduce violence:

- Resist pressure to hurt others or join gangs. Focus on your values and beliefs. Find healthy ways to feel good about yourself. Support others in resisting any pressure to act violently, too.
- Practice healthy conflict resolution. Use the negotiation process. Keep calm.
- Learn self-control and encourage others to use self-control.
- Choose your friends carefully. Build healthy relationships that are free from violence.
- Do not pick up a gun or other weapon. Report unsecure guns or weapons to a trusted adult.
- Be safe when home alone and in public places. For example, lock the doors and windows at home. Do not give out your personal information.
- If you are tempted to act violently, leave the situation. Seek help from a parent or other trusted adult.

Taking these steps can help build a safer community. Avoiding violence helps you and your community.

> **Essential Idea**
>
> To prevent violence, talk to a parent or other trusted adult if you are tempted to act violently or someone uses or threatens violence.

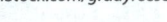

Figure 9.4.6 You can help reduce and prevent violence by behaving in a nonviolent way, standing up to violence, and practicing healthy conflict resolution.

9.4-6 Reading Checkpoint

1. Which three strategies to prevent and reduce violence do you think are most important for a young person to practice?
2. After reading this section, provide at least one question you now have or state one way this information can enhance your health or the health of others.

Lesson **9.4** **Review and Assessment**

Reading Summary

9.4–1 Any violent behavior that occurs in locations or events related to school is school violence.

9.4–2 Gang violence is carried out by groups of people who commit violent and illegal acts.

9.4–3 Human trafficking involves forcing people to perform a job or service against their will.

9.4–4 Threats or violence against someone because of race, ethnicity, disability, sex, or religion are hate crimes.

9.4–5 Killing someone is called homicide. It can be punished with life in prison, even for young people. The use of violence and threats to frighten or control groups of people is terrorism.

9.4–6 If you see or experience violence, tell a trusted adult. Get professional help for injuries. Practice healthy conflict resolution. Build healthy relationships free from violence.

Critical Thinking

1. **Explore.** What situations might increase the risk of community violence among young people? How can middle schoolers avoid these situations or react appropriately to them?
2. **Describe.** Why is it important to talk with a parent or other trusted adult and report any suspicious activity you see? How can you report these unsafe situations?

 Develop Your Skills

1. **Practice Health-Enhancing Behaviors and Set Goals.** Violence in communities is often outside of the control of middle school students. However, middle schoolers can do certain things to reduce their chances of being involved with violence. For example, being engaged in school activities and having strong social skills can decrease the risk of violence. Write a SMART goal for yourself that will help you reduce your risk of being involved in community violence.
2. **Advocate for Health.** Working in a team, review the information in this lesson about avoiding and preventing one type of community violence. Take notes and do additional research to learn about avoidance and prevention strategies. Design a poster or flyer that aims to reduce this type of violence in your community using the information from the chapter and additional resources. When creating your poster or flyer, keep in mind that you are providing information to middle school students. Make sure the material is appealing and appropriate for people your age.
3. **Access Information.** Many national organizations aim to end violence. Visit the website of one of these organizations. Is the information or service provided valid and reliable? How do you know? How accessible is the information or service to people in your community? Write a short summary outlining your answers.

Module 10 — Pregnancy and STIs

Lesson 10.1 Teen Pregnancy and Parenthood
Lesson 10.2 Sexually Transmitted Infections (STIs)
Lesson 10.3 HIV/AIDS

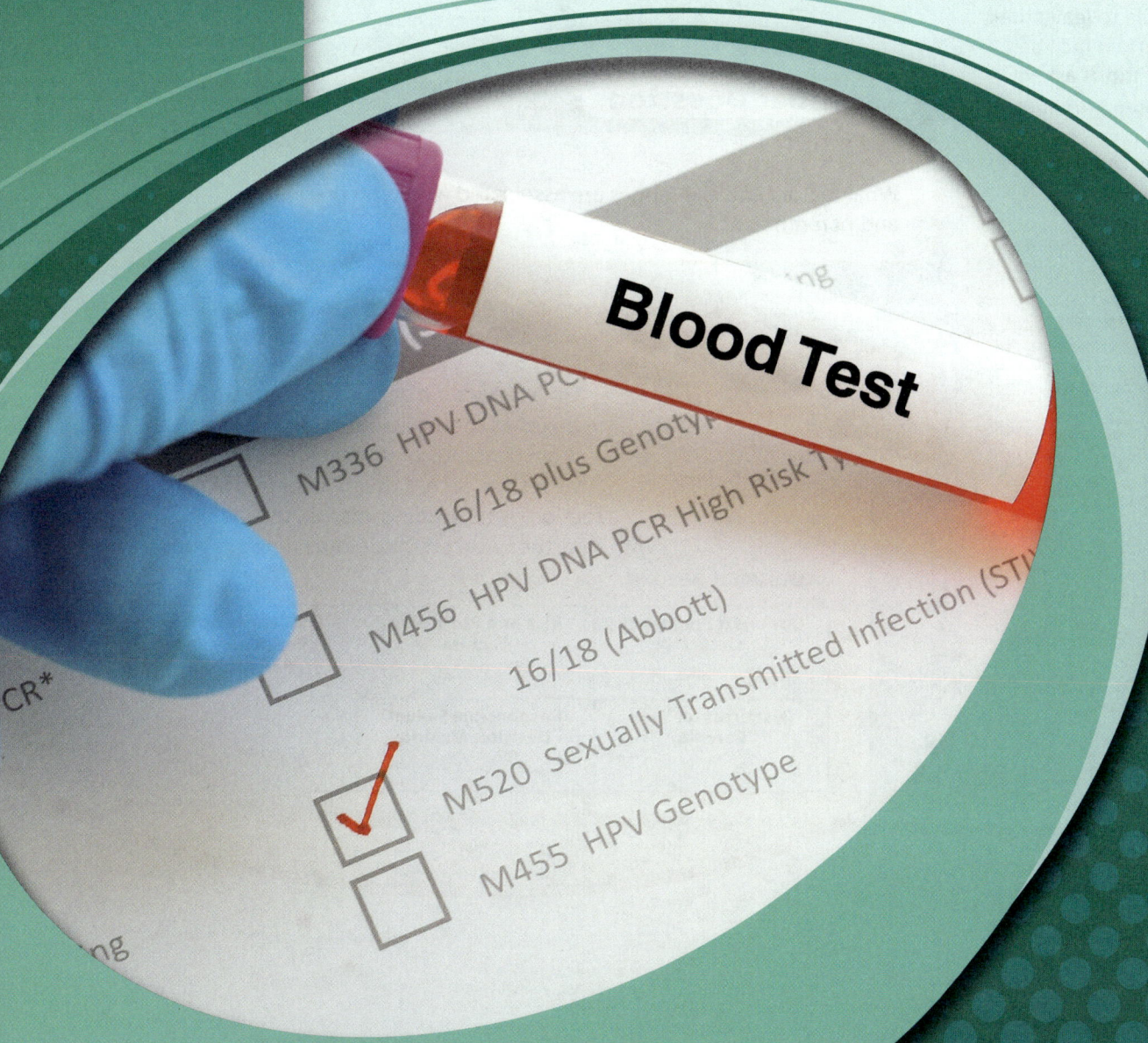

Jarun Ontakrai/Shutterstock.com

Lesson 10.1
Teen Pregnancy and Parenthood

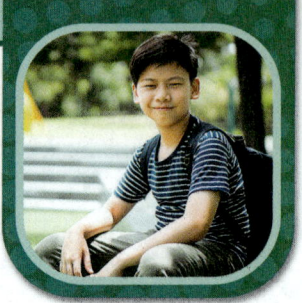

Key Terms

teen pregnancy pregnancy that occurs during the adolescent years when a person's body is still maturing and growing

teen parenthood act or process of teen parents raising a child

adoption action of legally raising another person's biological child

safe haven laws law that allows people to leave their babies at certain facilities with no questions asked; also called *safe surrender laws*

prenatal care medical care during pregnancy

Learning Outcomes

Look for the skills icon ✓ to practice health skills.
After studying this lesson, you will be able to

- **10.1-1 Recognize** different options for people who experience teen pregnancies.
- **10.1-2 List** risk and protective factors of teen pregnancy and parenthood.
- **10.1-3 Describe** the challenges of teen pregnancy and parenthood and how they can be managed.
- **10.1-4 Identify** resources for teen parents.
- **10.1-5 Implement** the decision-making process to help make responsible sexual decisions.

Essential Question

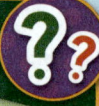

What factors and challenges are associated with teen pregnancy and parenthood?

Reading and Notetaking Activity

On a separate piece of paper, create five boxes as shown. Label each box with the main headings of the lesson. As you read the lesson, record the main points of each section. After reading, discuss the main points with a partner. Add any additional notes to your organizer as needed.

Options if Pregnancy Occurs	Risk and Protective Factors	Challenges of Teen Pregnancy and Parenthood
Resources for Teen Parents	Responsible Sexual Decision-Making	

Goodheart-Willcox Publisher

Lesson image: myboys.me/Shutterstock.com

Introduction

Ben knows that abstinence is a healthy sexual choice for young people to make. He knows other birth control methods can reduce the risk of pregnancy. He also knows pregnancies can still occur using these methods. Ben saw this firsthand when his older brother became a father in college. Ben loves his niece, but he does not want to have children until he has finished school.

Teen pregnancy is a pregnancy that occurs during the adolescent years. During this stage, a person's body is still maturing and growing. Knowing the facts about teen pregnancy and parenthood can help people make responsible decisions. For example, abstinence is the only 100 percent effective method of preventing pregnancy.

10.1-1 Options if Pregnancy Occurs

When pregnancy occurs, some teens choose to raise their child. With this choice, teens start the journey of **teen parenthood**.

If teens decide to parent their child, they must prepare and learn everything they can about parenthood. Parents are responsible for meeting all of the child's needs, such as food and shelter. They must also provide for the child's emotional and social needs.

Some teens may choose to place the child for *adoption* (Figure 10.1.1). In an **adoption**, a person legally raises another person's biological child. People choose adoption for a variety of reasons. People who choose this route may feel some grief and loss following adoption. However, this decision may be best for the well-being of the teen parent and their child. This choice can also help other couples have children.

Every state has **safe haven laws** (also called *safe surrender laws*). These laws allow people to leave their babies at certain facilities. If they do so, there will be no questions asked and no legal consequences. Babies will be well cared for until they can be adopted. These laws protect babies from the dangers of abandonment. Each state has age restrictions for a baby who is left at a safe haven. Safe havens include fire stations, police stations, and hospitals.

When considering their options, people can benefit from a strong family support system. Counseling from doctors and advisors can also be helpful.

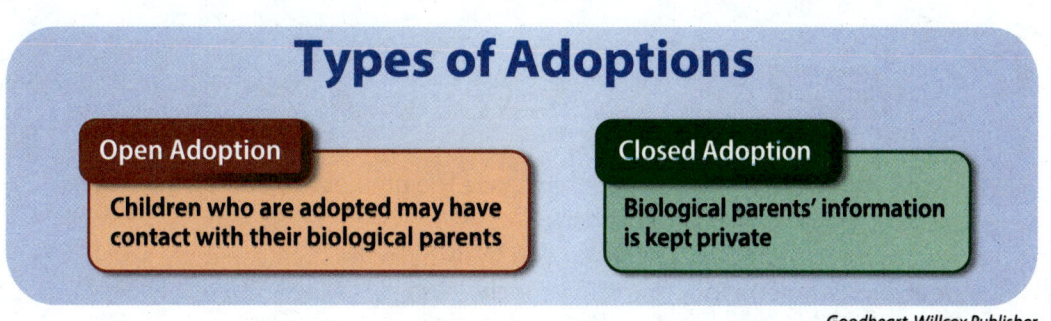

Figure 10.1.1 Adoption laws vary by state. People who choose to place a child for adoption have two options.

In which type of adoption is the biological parents' information kept private?

10.1–1 Reading Checkpoint

1. What are two options for a teen who becomes pregnant?
2. Describe safe haven laws. How do they impact teens?

10.1-2 Risk and Protective Factors

Essential Idea

Certain risk factors increase the risk for teen pregnancy, including limited knowledge of reproductive health, use of alcohol or drugs, and low self-esteem. Some factors, like parental or guardian support and continuous abstinence, can decrease the risk of teen pregnancy.

Several factors raise the risk for teen pregnancy. **Figure 10.1.2** lists examples of internal or external risk factors.

Protective factors decrease a person's chances of teen pregnancy and parenthood. Young people can build protective factors into their personal life. Examples of protective factors include the following parts of a person's life:

- discussion with parents, guardians, or healthcare professionals about reproductive health
- parental or guardian support and healthy family relationships
- healthy self-esteem
- support for mental and emotional health
- accurate knowledge of reproductive health
- continuous *abstinence*, or the commitment to refrain from sexual activity

Risk Factors for Teen Pregnancy and Parenthood

- Limited knowledge of reproductive health
- A parent who had a child before the age of 20
- Unprotected sexual activity
- Living in a home with frequent family conflict
- Use of alcohol or drugs
- Low self-esteem

Goodheart-Willcox Publisher

Figure 10.1.2 Risk factors for teen pregnancy and parenthood include a person's knowledge, choices, and environment.

10.1–2 Reading Checkpoint

1. Which three risk factors do you think have the greatest impact on a teen's risk of pregnancy? Explain your choices.
2. Which three protective factors do you think have the greatest impact on a teen's risk of pregnancy? Explain your choices.

10.1-3 Challenges of Teen Pregnancy and Parenthood

The challenges of pregnancy and parenthood may affect the physical, emotional, and social health of teen parents and their child. Teen parents may also face challenges to their education and finances (Figure 10.1.3).

Physical impacts of teen pregnancy can result from poor **prenatal care**, or medical care during pregnancy. Teen parents may neglect prenatal care. This can happen if they wish to keep a pregnancy secret. Some teens lack knowledge about proper prenatal care. Others may not know how to find or pay for prenatal care.

Poor prenatal care can harm the health of a teen who is pregnant. It can also harm the health of the fetus. For accurate information about prenatal care, teens can talk to a parent, guardian, other trusted adult, school nurse, or other medical professional.

People should never keep a pregnancy secret. Instead, they should visit a doctor to begin prenatal care as soon as possible. Prenatal care involves making regular visits to an obstetrician/gynecologist (OB/GYN). These doctors specialize in pregnancy, labor, and delivery. During pregnancy, people need to take special care of their own health. Doctors can advise people how to care for themselves and their fetus during pregnancy. General recommendations are included in Figure 10.1.4.

Emotions and feelings can overwhelm a teen parent. They may feel angry or depressed. This may happen as a teen realizes how pregnancy has altered their goals and futures. New challenges and responsibilities can cause them to feel stressed. Changes in hormones can lead to strong, unpredictable emotions for a pregnant person.

> **Essential Idea**
>
> Teen pregnancy may negatively impact teen parents as well as their children, families, and society. These impacts may be physical, social and emotional, financial, and educational.

Impacts of Teen Pregnancy and Parenthood

Area of Impact	Effects
Physical impacts	**Teen parents:** STIs from sexual intercourse, anemia, high blood pressure, childbirth complications (such as placenta previa, preeclampsia, premature delivery, and prolonged labor) **Child:** low birthweight, death within first year, dependence on addictive substances, slow growth, infections
Social and emotional impacts	**Teen parents:** Strained relationships with partner, friends, and family; anger and depression; disruption of life goals **Child:** Resentment from parents and stress can harm social and emotional health **Families:** Teen pregnancy can strain family relationships and cause stress **Society:** Family stress and conflict can cause stress in a community and society
Financial impacts	**Teen parents:** Too little money to cover expenses for the child **Child:** Financial strain to pay for necessities, more likely to have financial difficulties and become teen parents **Families:** Financial strain from caring for teen parents and the child **Society:** Social programs may help support teen parents and a child
Educational impacts	**Teen parents:** Disruption of education can lead to incomplete education and difficulty finding a job **Child:** Less likely to complete education **Families:** Childcare and expenses can disrupt other family members' educations **Society:** Teen pregnancy can lead to higher dropout rates and less education

Goodheart-Willcox Publisher

Figure 10.1.3 Teen parents, their children, their families, and society may face various challenges.

Figure 10.1.4 Consulting with a doctor can help pregnant people have a healthy pregnancy.

Healthy Behaviors of Pregnancy

Pregnant people *should*...	Pregnant people *should not*...
• tell a trusted adult about the pregnancy • begin prenatal care as soon as possible • take prenatal vitamins • get enough sleep each night • eat whole grains, fresh fruit, vegetables, and lean meats • drink plenty of water • take precautions to prevent STIs • get moderate physical activity	• keep pregnancy a secret • vape or smoke • drink alcohol • use drugs • eat an excessive amount of junk food • get excessive physical activity • diet to lose weight

Goodheart-Willcox Publisher

Costs of Raising a Child

Estimates of raising a child in the US range between $15,000 and $17,500 per year

- Housing
- Medical care
- Clothes and food
- Child care services
- Transportation

Goodheart-Willcox Publisher

Figure 10.1.5 The expenses for raising a child involve various items. Both parents are required to contribute.

How much is it estimated to cost to raise a child in the US per year?

Pregnancy can lead to changes, including stress and conflict, with a pregnant person's relationships friends, family, and dating partners. Pregnant teens and teen parents may have less time to spend hanging out with friends.

Teen parents can manage these social and emotional changes. They can take care of their mental and emotional health. Throughout pregnancy and parenthood, healthy relationships with family and friends are valuable resources. These relationships provide emotional support such as comfort, care, and encouragement. Family members can also assist with raising the child. Teens can also get professional help, if needed.

Teens may find it difficult to balance schoolwork with parenthood. It is important, however, for teen parents to complete their education. Earning at least a high school diploma leads to more chances for employment. A diploma helps parents provide financial support for their child (**Figure 10.1.5**).

Flexible options such as night classes or online courses may help busy parents complete their diploma. They may turn to family for support. Family members can help care for the child while the teen parents attend school or study. If family members are not available, the parents can seek child care services.

10.1–3 Reading Checkpoint

1. Summarize how pregnancy and parenthood can affect the physical, emotional, and social health of teens.
2. What challenges might the child of a teen parent face?

10.1-4 Resources for Teen Parents

New responsibilities can overwhelm or frustrate teens during pregnancy and parenthood. Teen parents are not alone when it comes to taking care of their child, however.

Numerous resources within a community can help teen parents (Figure 10.1.6). Teen parents can attend pregnancy and parenting support groups. This can help them understand how to meet the needs of raising a child. In support groups, teens meet other parents, share issues, and discuss solutions.

The government provides resources for teens who are pregnant or are parents. For example, Medicaid can assist teens with getting prenatal care.

One government resource is the *Special Supplemental Nutrition Program for Women, Infants, and Children (WIC)*. This program provides federal grants to states. These grants help pay for foods, healthcare referrals, and nutrition education. WIC provides assistance for pregnant people, parents who need financial help, and infants and children up to age five.

To make sure a resource is reliable and qualified, teens can check its background. To verify a resource's qualifications, search for answers to the following questions:

- **Is the resource licensed to operate for its stated purposes?** For example, a resource might have a license to provide counseling, prenatal care, or child care.
- **Do its professionals have credentials for their work?** Examples of credentials may include a professional degree, certification, or license.
- **Is the resource a non-profit or a profit-making group?** The main goal of a profit-making group is to make money by selling services or products. These groups may not serve the needs of teen parents.

Resources for Teen Parents and Families

- On-site child care in schools
- Babysitting through school or a community organization after school
- Personal and family counseling
- Career counseling
- Pregnancy and parenting support groups
- Parenting classes that teach the basics of care, feeding, sleeping, diapering, bathing, and child safety
- Online schooling and GED testing services

Goodheart-Willcox Publisher

Figure 10.1.6 Various resources exist for teen parents and their families within a community to help with raising a child.

10.1-4 Reading Checkpoint

1. Describe resources that are available for teen parents. How can these resources have a positive impact on the health of a teen parent and their child?
2. How can a young person check that a resource is reliable and qualified?

10.1-5 Responsible Sexual Decision-Making

Making healthy sexual decisions can be difficult for young people. They may feel pressured by peers, partners, or the media. The decision-making process can help young people make these decisions. For example, Figure 10.1.7 shows an example of how to use this process to practice abstinence.

Young people are still growing and maturing. Practicing continuous abstinence and refusal skills gives them time to mature before starting a sexual relationship. Doing proper research and asking parents, guardians, or other trusted adults questions can also help young people make safe sexual decisions.

Figure 10.1.7 The decision-making process can be used to help young people make healthy sexual choices.

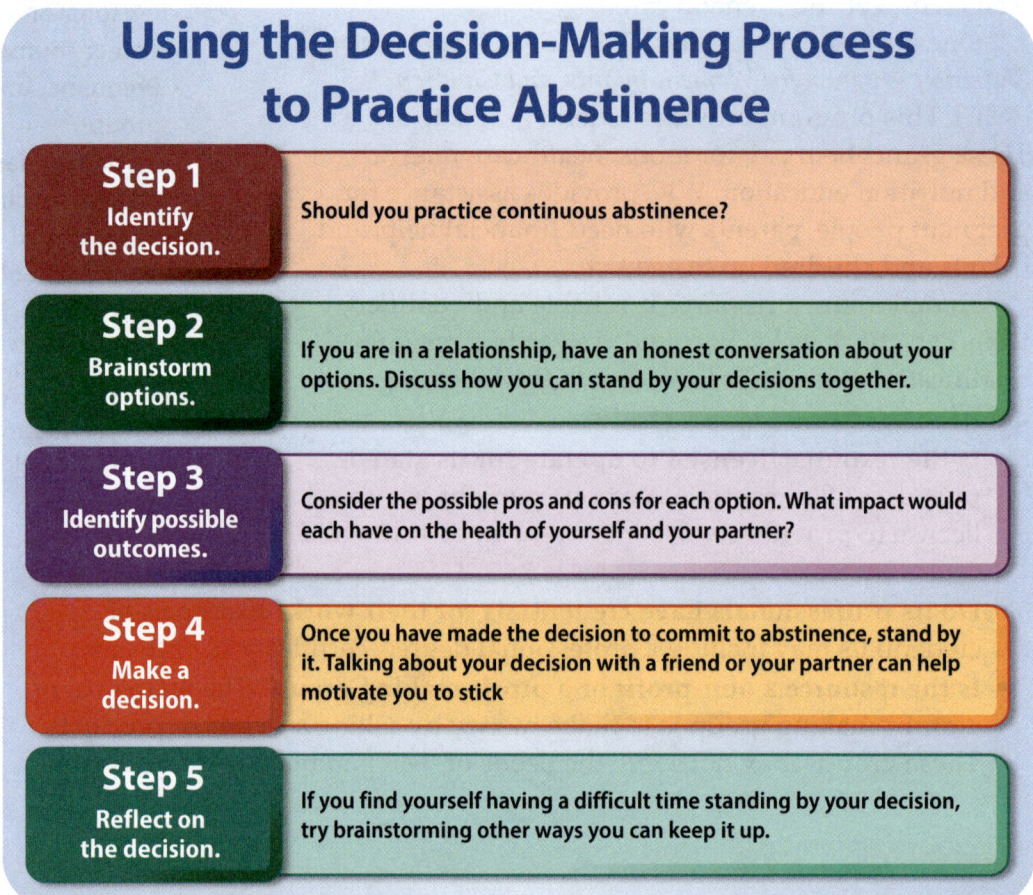

Using the Decision-Making Process to Practice Abstinence

Step 1 Identify the decision.
Should you practice continuous abstinence?

Step 2 Brainstorm options.
If you are in a relationship, have an honest conversation about your options. Discuss how you can stand by your decisions together.

Step 3 Identify possible outcomes.
Consider the possible pros and cons for each option. What impact would each have on the health of yourself and your partner?

Step 4 Make a decision.
Once you have made the decision to commit to abstinence, stand by it. Talking about your decision with a friend or your partner can help motivate you to stick

Step 5 Reflect on the decision.
If you find yourself having a difficult time standing by your decision, try brainstorming other ways you can keep it up.

Goodheart-Willcox Publisher

BUILDING YOUR SKILLS — Mental Health Connections

Making Decisions About Boundaries

As a young person, you might be in a dating relationship already. You might be thinking about the possibility of a new dating relationship. You might also have no interest in dating yet. Young people develop an interest in dating at different rates and all are normal.

Regardless of your experiences with dating, it is important to begin to think about your expectations and boundaries in a dating relationship. Certain factors, such as peer pressure, media influence, and substance use, may impact your decisions about sexual activity. Ultimately, however, this decisions are up to you. Creating boundaries can help you be more in control of your body and decisions.

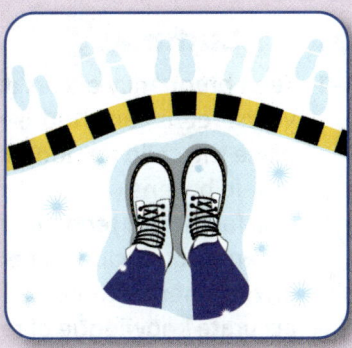

Ok Sotnikova/Shutterstock.com

✓ Practice Your Skills — Advocate for Health

Reflect on your expectations and boundaries in a dating relationship. Create a personal message that states your boundaries. This message can be in the form of a letter, blog, vlog, one-pager, or other creative product. Once complete, share your message with at least one person in your life (parent, guardian, other trusted adult, best friend, sibling, etc.) and begin the conversation about responsible sexual decisions.

10.1–5 Reading Checkpoint

1. Why is choosing abstinence and practicing refusal skills the healthiest choice for young people?
2. Do you think most young people use all the steps in the decision-making process to make responsible health decisions? Defend your answer.

Lesson 10.1 Review and Assessment

Reading Summary

10.1–1 Teen pregnancy occurs during the adolescent years. Teens can choose teen parenthood, place the child for adoption, or leave the baby at safe havens.

10.1–2 Risk factors for teen pregnancy and parenthood include a person's choices and environment. Protective factors include accurate knowledge of reproductive health and continuous abstinence.

10.1–3 Challenges of teen pregnancy and parenthood can affect the well-being of teen parents, as well as their child.

10.1–4 Resources for teen parents include prenatal care, healthy relationships, completing education, and community and government resources.

10.1–5 Knowing how to make responsible sexual decisions that reflect your goals can help with your overall physical, mental and emotional, and social health.

Critical Thinking

1. **Explain.** What can your school and community do to encourage responsible sexual decision-making among young people?
2. **Predict.** How would your life change if you found out today that you were going to be a parent?

Develop Your Skills

1. **Communicate with Others.** Imagine that you have a friend who is considering becoming sexually active. Your friend knows that sexual activity could lead to pregnancy but thinks it is unlikely to happen and believes that raising a child would not be that difficult. Using the information you learned in this lesson, write a letter to your friend outlining how teen pregnancy and parenthood can change a person's life. Recommend abstinence in the letter. Then, divide into small groups to discuss your letters and ways to make them more effective.
2. **Set Goals.** Decide on four important goals you have for your future. Now, imagine that you are about to become an adolescent parent. You have made the decision to raise the child. What effect will your decision to be an adolescent parent have on your future goals? Write a personal reflection including the following information: List each goal and describe how teen parenthood will affect it. Next, reflect on how you would adjust your goals to be successful at both teen parenthood and your personal goals.
3. **Make Decisions.** Read the following scenario: *Sarah just found out that she is pregnant. As a teen, she is overwhelmed, confused, and scared. She has no idea how to tell her partner and parents. She wonders how long she can hide the pregnancy. Feeling alone, she reflects on all her options.* With a partner, list at least three options and the pros and cons of each option. Based on the pros and cons of each option, decide on the best course of action. Defend your decision.

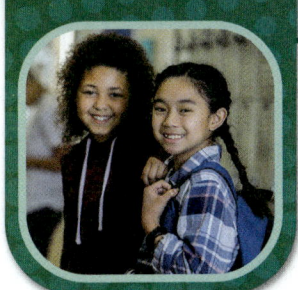

Sexually Transmitted Infections (STIs)

Lesson **10.2**

Learning Outcomes

Look for the skills icon ✓ to practice health skills.
After studying this lesson, you will be able to

- **10.2-1 Understand** how people contract sexually transmitted infections (STIs).
- **10.2-2 Describe** the most commonly reported STIs.
- **10.2-3 Identify** methods for preventing STIs.
- **10.2-4 Explain** treatment methods and resources for STIs.

Essential Question

What are common STIs and how can they be prevented and treated?

Reading and Notetaking Activity

As you read or listen to your teacher present this lesson, use an organizer to visually organize your notes about the most common STIs. Identify whether the cause of the STI is a bacterium, virus, or protozoa. Then, identify the effects and possible treatments for each STI.

Chlamydia Cause: Health effects: Treatment:	**Genital Herpes** Cause: Health effects: Treatment:
Gonorrhea Cause: Health effects: Treatment:	**Human papillomavirus (HPV)** Cause: Health effects: Treatment:
Syphilis Cause: Health effects: Treatment:	**Hepatitis** Cause: Health effects: Treatment:
Trichomoniasis Cause: Health effects: Treatment:	

Goodheart-Willcox Publisher

Key Terms

sexually transmitted infections (STIs) infectious diseases spread from one person to another primarily through sexual activity

chlamydia bacterial infection known as a "silent" disease because it has few or no symptoms

gonorrhea bacterial infection that mainly affects the genitals, rectum, and throat

syphilis bacterial infection that develops in stages and causes extremely serious health conditions

trichomoniasis curable infection caused by protozoa

genital herpes viral infection that causes sores on the genitals, mouth, or rectum

human papillomavirus (HPV) most commonly contracted STI; causes genital infections and may cause cancer

hepatitis potentially severe liver disease caused by different viruses

condom device that provides a barrier to pathogens that cause STIs

Lesson image:
Courtney Hale/E+ via Getty Images

Introduction

Sexually transmitted infections (STIs) are infectious diseases that spread from one person to another primarily through sexual activity. Sometimes, STIs are called *sexually transmitted diseases (STDs)*.

According to the World Health Organization (WHO), more than one million STIs are contracted each day around the world (Figure 10.2.1). STIs can affect people of any biological sex, age, race, nationality, and ethnic origin.

Figure 10.2.1 Of the commonly reported STIs, the most frequent is HPV.

Most commonly reported STIs
- Chlamydia
- Gonorrhea
- Syphilis
- Trichomoniasis
- Genital herpes
- Human papillomavirus (HPV)

Goodheart-Willcox Publisher

10.2-1 How People Contract STIs

Just as with other infectious diseases, bacteria, viruses, and protozoa cause STIs. These pathogens live in and on the surfaces of the reproductive organs. For some STIs, the pathogens may also live in the mouth, rectum, blood, and other bodily fluids.

STIs spread mainly through *sexual activity*. This can include sexual touching and sexual intercourse. These actions involve skin-to-skin contact with a person's external reproductive organs and the exchange of bodily fluids.

Engaging in sexual activity just one time with just one person who has an STI is all it takes to contract an STI. People with more sexual partners have greater risk of getting an STI.

Certain *oral* (appearing on the mouth) STIs may spread by kissing, but other STIs are not transmitted this way. Casual contact, such as using the same toilet seat, does not transmit STIs.

Some methods outside of sexual activity can transmit an STI. For example, a pregnant person can transmit syphilis to the fetus. Chlamydia can be transmitted to the newborn during childbirth. People can contract an STI when using infected needles to inject drugs.

10.2–1 Reading Checkpoint

1. How are STIs spread?
2. Based on how STIs are spread, do you think young people are at risk of contracting an STI? Defend your answer.

10.2–2 Common STIs

As you read the following sections, you will learn about the signs, symptoms, and treatments for common STIs.

Chlamydia

Chlamydia is a common STI, caused by bacteria, that is a "silent" disease because it often has few or no symptoms. Due to its lack of symptoms, the CDC reports that more than one million cases of chlamydia go undiagnosed each year.

When symptoms occur, they are often mild. People may feel nausea or a burning sensation during urination. Chlamydia is a serious threat to female reproductive health. As a silent disease, it can quietly become a serious infection of the internal female reproductive organs. This condition, called *pelvic inflammatory disease (PID)*, can cause *infertility*, or the inability to become pregnant. PID also raises the risk for cancer of the ovaries.

Trichomoniasis

Trichomoniasis is an infection caused by protozoa. As many as 70 percent of people with trichomoniasis do not show any signs or symptoms. This can cause the infection to go undiagnosed and untreated and people can then infect their sexual partners. When symptoms do occur, trichomoniasis mostly causes itching, burning, and pain during urination in the female reproductive system.

Gonorrhea

Gonorrhea is a bacterial infection that mainly affects the genitals, rectum, and throat. According to the CDC, gonorrhea is a very common STI among people between 15 and 24 years of age. Like chlamydia, gonorrhea often causes few or no symptoms. In some cases of gonorrhea, however, symptoms do develop (**Figure 10.2.2**).

Essential Idea

Common STIs include chlamydia, trichomoniasis, gonorrhea, syphilis, genital herpes, human papillomavirus, and hepatitis.

Figure 10.2.2 Many cases of gonorrhea present few or no symptoms. The symptoms that do develop vary between the male and female reproductive systems.

Is pelvic and lower back pain a symptom of gonorrhea in the male or female reproductive system?

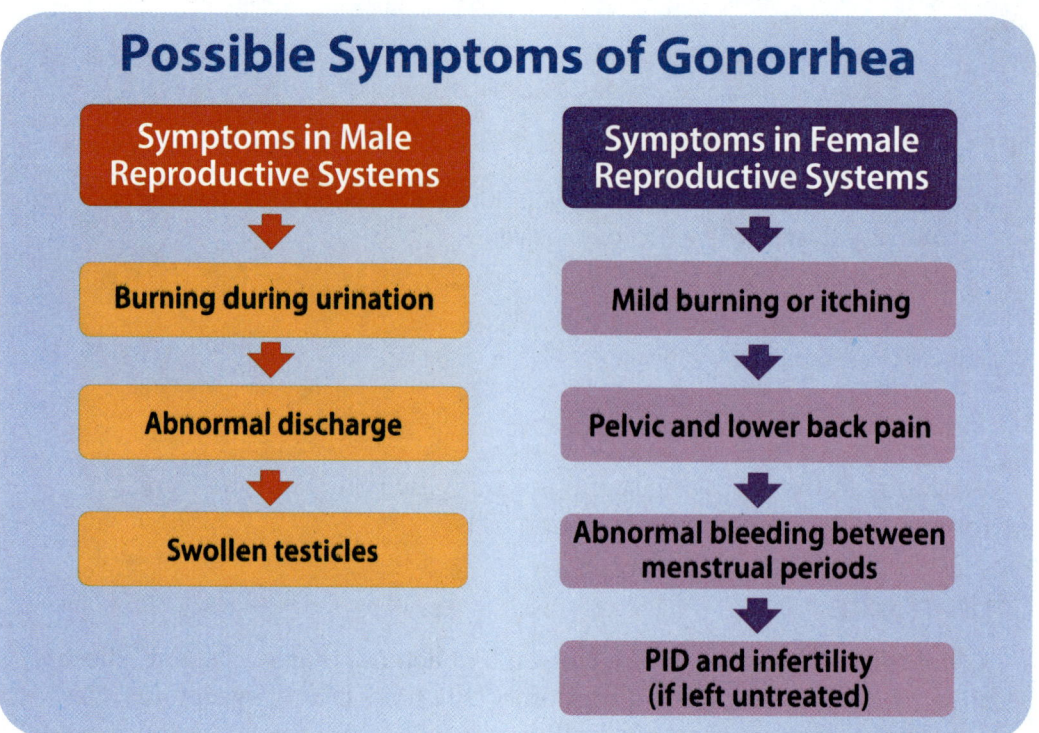

Syphilis

Syphilis is a bacterial infection that can cause serious health conditions. This STI develops in stages, which include the following:

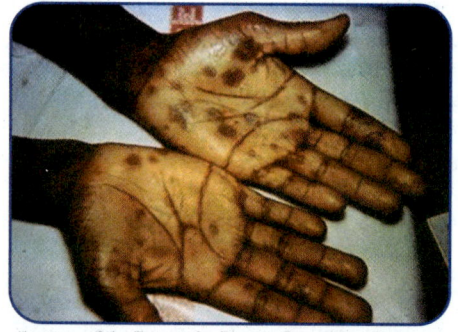

Courtesy of the Centers for Disease Control and Prevention

Figure 10.2.3 A syphilis rash often appears on the palms of the hands and soles of the feet, but sometimes elsewhere.

- **Primary syphilis.** During this first stage, sores develop at the site of the infection. Direct contact with a syphilis sore during sexual activity spreads syphilis. The sores are not painful, do not itch, and heal after a few weeks.
- **Secondary syphilis.** The second stage develops days, weeks, or even months after the primary stage. In this stage, a red or copper-color rash appears (Figure 10.2.3). The rash heals, but the person still has syphilis.
- **Latent syphilis.** During the latent stage, a person still has syphilis, but there are no signs or symptoms of the disease.
- **Late-stage syphilis.** This final stage is an internal disease. This stage often causes no obvious external signs. Damage to the brain leads to a type of *dementia* (loss of mental function) and paralysis. Late-stage syphilis also causes fatal damage to the heart, liver, and blood vessels.

Genital Herpes

Genital herpes is a viral STI that causes sores on the genitals, mouth, or rectum. Two types of herpes simplex virus (HSV) cause genital herpes: *HSV type 1* and *HSV type 2* (Figure 10.2.4). Genital herpes is very common in the United States among people between 14 and 49 years of age.

A person with genital herpes often has mild or no symptoms at first. Eventually, blisters arise at the site of infection. The blisters burst and heal

Herpes Simplex Viruses That Cause Genital Herpes

HSV-1
- Cold sores on mouth and lips and genital infections
- Transmitted by kissing or through sexual activity

HSV-2
- Genital infections only
- Transmitted only through sexual contact

Goodheart-Willcox Publisher

Figure 10.2.4 The two types of herpes viruses are spread by different kinds of direct contact. These viruses cause different infections. *Which type of HSV causes genital infections only?*

after a few weeks. These blisters often return, but in a milder form. Sometimes, people develop swollen lymph nodes and fever. This return of genital herpes is called an outbreak. Genital herpes can also lead to infertility.

Human Papillomavirus

Human papillomavirus (HPV) is the most commonly contracted STI. HPV infects cells in skin and membranes, causing them to grow abnormally. At least 40 kinds of HPV can cause genital infections. Some types can cause cancer.

Almost all sexually active people carry HPV at one time or another. Luckily, the body fights and eliminates most HPV infections. Some types of HPV, however, cause genital warts or cervical cancer (Figure 10.2.5). HPV can also cause cancer of the penis, mouth, and throat. HPV infections can lead to infertility.

Hepatitis

Hepatitis is a potentially severe liver disease caused by different hepatitis viruses. Hepatitis A, B, and C are three hepatitis viruses that can be transmitted by sexual activity, among other methods, including contaminated food and water and sharing contaminated needles.

Growths Caused by HPV

Genital Warts
- Abnormal growths on the skin and membranes around the genitals, mouth, and rectum
- Range from small raised bumps to large cauliflower shapes

Cervical Cancer
- Abnormal cancerous growth of the cervix
- Affects the female reproductive system

Goodheart-Willcox Publisher

Figure 10.2.5 The body fights and eliminates most types of HPV. Some types of HPV, however, can cause genital warts or cervical cancer.

Hepatitis A is usually a short-term illness. Most people can recover fully. A few weeks or months after the liver becomes infected, toxins and waste build up in the blood. These cause yellow skin or eyes. They can also cause nausea, appetite loss, vomiting, fever, and fatigue.

Hepatitis B and C may have short-term and severe long-term effects. Many people have short-term illnesses. Some people develop liver cancer or permanent liver damage called *cirrhosis*.

10.2–2 Reading Checkpoint

1. Choose two common STIs and describe their symptoms.
2. How is it possible for a young person to have an STI and not know they have it?

CASE STUDY

Aiden's "Perfect" Relationship

Bryan has always looked up to his older brother Aiden. Aiden taught him to throw a baseball, lift weights, and play video games. He seemed invincible—until recently.

Bryan adored Aiden's girlfriend, Ellie. They seemed perfect for each other. Together, they all played soccer and enjoyed working out. Ellie and Aiden often helped Bryan with his homework. Then, one day, Ellie stopped coming over and Aiden seemed distant and angry. After one week, Aiden confessed to Bryan what was happening. Aiden

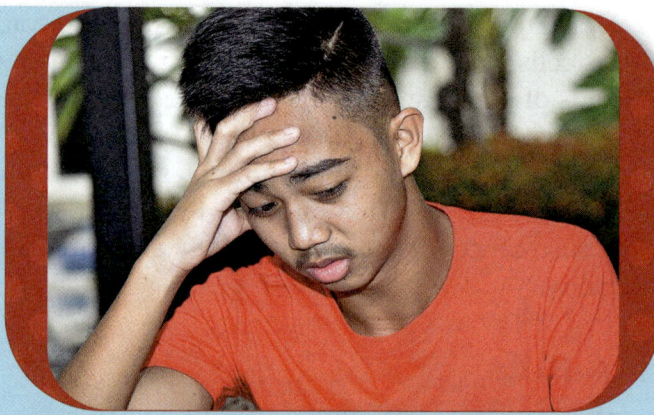

cheapbooks/Shutterstock.com

had developed swollen testicles and he felt burning when he urinated. Hoping for answers, Aiden had turned to Ellie, but she was argumentative and defensive.

 Practice Your Skills **Communicate with Others**

Bryan recently learned about STIs and the importance of getting tested and treated. With a partner, role play a conversation between Bryan and Aiden. Using empathy and supportive words, Bryan should initiate a conversation about STIs, the importance of getting tested, support from family members, and the benefits of abstinence. Switch roles so both partners have an opportunity to be Bryan in the conversation.

102 Module Pregnancy and STIs

10.2-3 Preventing STIs

Although treatments exist for STIs, it is easier to prevent STIs than it is to treat them. Three of the most effective methods for preventing STIs include sexual abstinence, the use of condoms, and vaccines.

Practicing Abstinence

The most effective way to prevent STIs is to practice sexual abstinence. *Sexual abstinence* is the commitment to refrain from sexual activity. Abstinence is the only 100 percent effective method for preventing STIs.

Barriers such as peer pressure may discourage people from practicing abstinence. These barriers may also keep people from setting boundaries and respecting others' limits. Friends or partners may try to persuade a person to engage in sexual activity. This is negative peer pressure. However, positive peer pressure can help people set and respect boundaries.

The use of alcohol and drugs can impair judgment. Alcohol and drugs lower a person's *inhibition* (feelings of restraint). Reduced inhibition can lead to early or unwanted sexual activity. Avoiding risky situations that may involve drugs and alcohol helps a person stick to their choice to stay abstinent.

Committing to abstinence may require a person to use refusal skills. Refusal skills can help someone stand up to peer pressure. Planning and practicing these skills can help prepare people to use words and actions if risky situations occur (**Figure 10.2.6**).

> **Essential Idea**
>
> Abstinence is the only 100 percent effective method for preventing STIs. The use of condoms and vaccines can also prevent STIs.

Planning and Practicing Refusal Skills

Practice
- Before you are presented with a risky situation, consider the words you might use.
- What if you are invited to an unsupervised party where alcohol or drugs may be present?
- What if your dating partner is pressuring you to have sex?

Refuse
- Verbally refuse the risky behavior. Be assertive and honest. Keep your response short, clear, and simple.
- If verbally refusing is not enough, walk away from the situation.

Seek Advice
- Remember that you do not need to face this stress alone.
- Find guidance for handling specific situations from a parent, teacher, counselor, or other trusted adult.

Goodheart-Willcox Publisher

Figure 10.2.6 Preparing your refusal skills in advance can help you be ready to deal with negative peer pressures.

Using Condoms

While not 100 percent effective, a correctly used condom can reduce the risk of contracting STIs. A **condom** is a device that provides a barrier to pathogens that cause STIs. Condoms may be external or internal. An *external condom* fits over an erect penis. An *internal condom* fits inside the vagina. External and internal condoms should *not* be used together.

Most condoms are made of latex. Using a latex condom helps prevent STI transmission. Condoms made of polyurethane or polyisoprene also prevent STI transmission. Condoms made of natural materials (for example, *lambskin condoms*) do not help prevent STIs. This is because they contain tiny holes through which pathogens can pass.

Condoms are still risky because they may fail. A person must never use a condom that has expired, has holes or tears, or has dried out. These condoms will not work. Condoms may become damaged if stored in places that become very cold or hot, such as in a car. They can be damaged if stored in a wallet, where they could be crushed. Condoms should be obtained from a reliable source, such as a clinic nurse, or from a store.

Condoms only cover the skin on the penis. STIs can still be transmitted through contact with other infected skin surfaces.

Vaccines

A vaccine can reduce the risk for an STI. For help making decisions about vaccines, talk to your parent or guardian and a healthcare professional.

The HPV vaccine has reduced HPV transmission by 86 percent among female teens in the US. The vaccine is recommended for people from 11 to 12 years of age. The vaccine is given in three shots over a six-month period. If people do not get the entire vaccine at this age, they can still receive the vaccine between 13 and 26 years of age.

A vaccine can also prevent hepatitis A and B. These vaccines are effective at preventing infection. People should get the vaccine if traveling to areas where hepatitis A is common. The hepatitis B vaccine is usually given to infants.

10.2–3 Reading Checkpoint

1. Why might abstinence be a challenge for some young people?
2. How might a condom not protect against STIs?
3. Besides abstinence and condoms, what is another way to prevent some STIs?

10.2-4 Treatment of STIs

Treatment is more effective for early stages of many STIs. For this reason, sexually active people should get regular tests for STIs. They should also get tested if they develop signs or symptoms of an STI (Figure 10.2.7).

Trichomoniasis may be the most curable of the common STIs. It is easily cured with prescription medications. It is important, however, for all partners to be treated, even if they do not show any symptoms. Treatments for other STIs depend on whether they are caused by bacteria or viruses.

Bacterial STIs

Bacterial STIs are treatable, even curable, with antibiotics prescribed by a doctor.

- **Chlamydia.** Chlamydia can be treated and cured with prescription antibiotics.
- **Gonorrhea.** Doctors often prescribe two kinds of antibiotics to treat and cure gonorrhea.
- **Syphilis.** Antibiotics may treat and cure syphilis in its primary and secondary stages. Even if late-term syphilis is cured, organ damage remains permanent.

> **Essential Idea**
>
> Trichomoniasis can be treated and cured with medications. Bacterial STIs can be treated with antibiotics. Antiviral medicines can reduce how severely and frequently people experience the symptoms of viral STIs.

Sexually Transmitted Infections

Name	Symptoms
Chlamydia	• Vaginal or penile discharge, painful urination, fever • If left untreated, may damage reproductive organs and cause infertility
Gonorrhea	• Vaginal or penile discharge, painful or frequent urination, fever, abdominal pain • If left untreated, may damage reproductive organs and cause infertility
Syphilis	• Early stage: small, painless sore on affected area • Later stages: body rash, fever, hair and weight loss, headache, sore muscles • If left untreated, may cause permanent internal damage and death
Trichomoniasis	• For males: itching and burning in the urethra, discharge from the penis • For females: yellow-green vaginal discharge with a foul odor, burning, itching, and pain during urination and sexual intercourse
Genital herpes	• Blisters or sores around the affected area with pain and itching
HPV	• Warts on genitals, painful urination • Cervical and other types of cancer
Hepatitis	• For hepatitis A: yellow skin or eyes, nausea, appetite loss, vomiting, fever, fatigue • For hepatitis B and C: short-term illnesses, liver cancer, or permanent liver damage (*cirrhosis*)

Goodheart-Willcox Publisher

Figure 10.2.7 While it is possible that an STI will not show any noticeable symptoms, most STIs show some symptoms.

Which STI triggers hair and weight loss in later stages?

BUILDING YOUR SKILLS: Community Connections

Testing and Treatment

Young people often do not know where to go to ask questions about their reproductive health, not to mention seeking testing or treatment for an STI. Some young people feel comfortable asking their parents or guardians questions. Others would rather talk to another trusted adult.

Fortunately, many community resources can help young people trying to take care of their reproductive health. Public health departments, private and nonprofit organizations, doctors' offices, and even some schools offer resources to help educate young people about reproductive health and STIs. Some of these resources may also offer testing and treatment.

Learning about these community resources can help you remember them if you ever do have questions about your reproductive health or need to get testing or treatment for an STI.

tulpahn/Shutterstock.com

Practice Your Skills: Access Information

Do you know what resources are available to educate young people and provide STI testing and treatment in your community? In this activity, you will identify these resources and keep a list for your future reference.

To identify community resources, do research using valid and reliable sources. You can also talk with a parent, guardian, other trusted adult, or school nurse. The community resources you identify should support reproductive health, answer reproductive health questions, educate people about ways to prevent STIs, and provide treatment options.

Collect the following information for three or more resources in your community: name of the resource, contact information, and services provided. Create a graphic or visual to organize your information.

Being cured, however, does not mean that people cannot contract bacterial STIs again. Even after receiving treatment, exposure to an STI will result in another infection.

Some strains of bacteria have adapted to antibiotics used to treat them. For example, some returning gonorrhea infections are more difficult to treat. These strains cause more serious disease that lasts longer.

Viral STIs

Viral STIs cannot be cured, but antiviral medicines can reduce how severely and frequently people experience the symptoms.

- **Genital herpes.** Prescribed medication can control breakouts and symptoms of genital herpes.
- **HPV.** If a person develops genital warts from an HPV infection, a doctor may prescribe skin treatments, medication, or surgical removal. Treatments for cancer caused by HPV depend on the nature of each cancer.

- **Hepatitis A.** For most people, hepatitis A can be treated with rest, fluids, and good nutrition. People with severe symptoms may need care in a hospital.
- **Hepatitis B.** People who have been exposed to hepatitis B can receive antibody injections.
- **Hepatitis C.** Hepatitis C can be treated with medication taken over eight to 12 weeks.

STI Resources

Community resources can help people who suspect they might have an STI. Doctors can provide tests to determine whether someone has an STI. They can also prescribe treatment if necessary. Under certain circumstances, minors have access to STI testing and treatment in all 50 states.

County, state, or federal sources provide reliable information about STIs. Public health clinics often provide diagnosis, treatment, and prevention programs. Private and nonprofit organizations may also offer assistance or online testing. Some schools may provide reproductive health programs.

Having an STI can be stressful or scary. Those who need emotional support may find counseling services and support groups in their communities. People may also find support through their friends and family.

A parent or other trusted adult can help people locate the testing or treatment they need. People can learn more about resources available to them by searching the internet or by asking a doctor or nurse. Getting help when necessary is a good way to promote overall health and well-being.

10.2-4 Reading Checkpoint

1. What treatments can be used to treat trichomoniasis, viral STIs, and bacterial STIs?
2. When and where should a person get tested for an STI?

Lesson 10.2 Review and Assessment

Reading Summary

10.2–1 Sexually transmitted infections (STIs) are communicable diseases that spread from one person to another mainly during sexual activity. They are caused by pathogens.

10.2–2 Common STIs include chlamydia, gonorrhea, syphilis, trichomoniasis, genital herpes, human papillomavirus (HPV), and hepatitis.

10.2–3 Sexual abstinence, or refraining from sexual activity, is the only 100 percent effective method for preventing STIs. Using a latex condom during sexual activity can also reduce a person's risk of contracting an STI. Some vaccines can also prevent transmission of STIs

10.2–4 Some STIs are easily treated and curable, and others are not. People can receive STI testing from doctors, public health departments, and organizations offering in-person or online services.

Critical Thinking

1. **Determine.** What is the impact of contracting an STI?
2. **Conclude.** Who do you think is responsible for educating young people on STIs and the community resources available to support their health?

Develop Your Skills

1. **Access Information and Make Decisions.** The HPV vaccine is recommended for people from 11 to 12 years of age. Research several valid and reliable sources to learn more about the HPV vaccine. Record the pros and cons to getting the vaccine and other relevant information you learned from your research. Based on your initial research, who do you think should decide to get the vaccine? Would you consider getting the vaccine yourself? What questions do you have for your parent or guardian and doctor?
2. **Analyze Influences.** Reflect on how the media portrays dating relationships among young people. For those relationships that include sexual activity, how are STIs addressed? Create a mind map or graphic organizer to compile your thoughts. Based on your findings, write a short essay on the following topic: Does the media educate young people on responsible sexual decisions and STI prevention, testing, and treatment? What could the media do differently to have a more positive impact?
3. **Advocate for Health.** In small groups, write a message that educates on ways to prevent STIs, encourages abstinence, and identifies community resources and trusted adults who can support reproductive health. Turn your message into a product such as a flyer, poster, or public service announcement. With your teacher's permission, share your product with other students at your school.

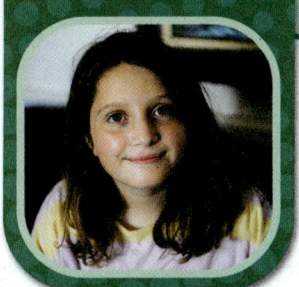

HIV/AIDS

Lesson **10.3**

Learning Outcomes

Look for the skills icon ✓ *to practice health skills.*
After studying this lesson, you will be able to

10.3–1 **Understand** the transmission methods, signs, and symptoms of HIV/AIDS.
10.3–2 **Explain** testing procedures for diagnosing HIV.
10.3–3 **Identify** treatment methods for HIV/AIDS.
10.3–4 **List** strategies for preventing HIV/AIDS.

Essential Question

What are HIV and AIDS and how can people prevent and treat them?

Reading and Notetaking Activity

Create a KWL chart. Before you read the lesson, outline what you know and what you want to know about understanding HIV/AIDS. After reading the lesson, outline what you have learned.

K: What I Know
- HIV infects and kills cells, weakening the body's immune system.
-

W: What I Want to Know
- Does everyone infected with HIV develop AIDS?
-

L: What I Have Learned
- AIDS is a condition in which the body cannot fight infections/disease; can develop later after HIV onset.
-

Goodheart-Willcox Publisher

Key Terms

human immunodeficiency virus (HIV) bloodborne virus that infects and kills white blood cells, weakening the body's immune system; can lead to AIDS

acquired immunodeficiency syndrome (AIDS) health condition in which the body cannot fight infections

long-term non-progressors people living with HIV whose infection progresses to AIDS very slowly

opportunistic infections conditions that occur when pathogens take advantage of a weakened immune system; the cause of death in HIV/AIDS cases

antiretroviral therapy (ART) treatment for HIV/AIDS in which a combination of drugs is given to control HIV reproduction in the body

pre-exposure prophylaxis (PrEP) type of ART that helps prevent HIV transmission; comes in a pill taken daily

post-exposure prophylaxis (PEP) emergency type of ART that a person can take after potential exposure to HIV to reduce risk of transmission

Lisa5201/iStock/Getty Images Plus via Getty Images

Introduction

Around the world, more than 38 million people are living with HIV/AIDS. Since this epidemic began, the World Health Organization (WHO) estimates 40 million people have died from AIDS-related causes.

HIV/AIDS affects people of any biological sex, age, race, nationality, and ethnic origin. HIV transmission is most common among people ages 13–34.

In this lesson, you will learn about what HIV/AIDS is. You will also learn about the transmission and signs and symptoms of HIV/AIDS. Finally, you will learn about testing, preventing, and treating HIV/AIDS.

10.3-1 Understanding HIV and AIDS

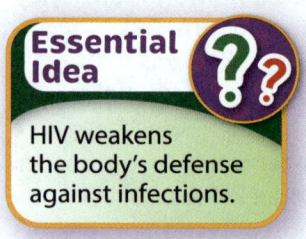

Essential Idea

HIV weakens the body's defense against infections.

To understand HIV and AIDS, you must first know what each term means (Figure 10.3.1). **Human immunodeficiency virus (HIV)** infects and kills white blood cells, weakening the body's immune system. At a certain point, HIV can completely wear down the immune system. This leads to **acquired immunodeficiency syndrome (AIDS)**, a health condition in which the body cannot fight infections.

AIDS can develop later, perhaps many years after the onset of HIV. Treatment can slow the progression of HIV into AIDS and help people with AIDS live longer. Many people who have HIV/AIDS can live long, healthy lives if they receive regular treatment. Treatment also greatly reduces the risk for HIV transmission.

A positive test for HIV detects the presence of HIV *antibodies* in the person's blood. *Antibodies* are proteins the body's immune system produces to detect

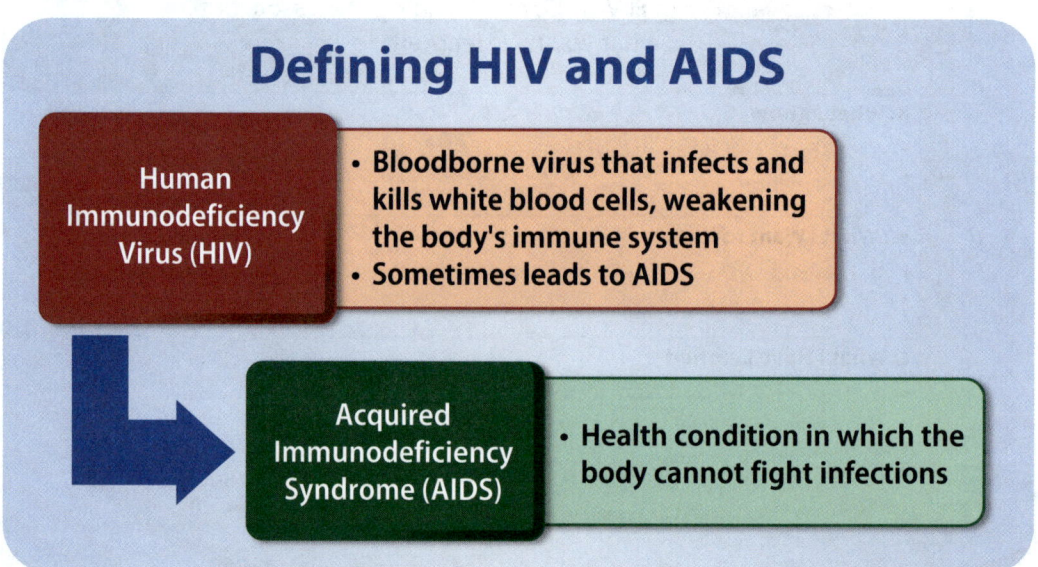

Figure 10.3.1 HIV is a virus that infects cells and weakens the body's immune system. Sometimes, perhaps many years after the onset of HIV, a person can develop AIDS, in which the body cannot fight infections.

Which health condition can sometimes come from HIV?

and destroy certain harmful substances, such as HIV. If HIV antibodies are in a person's blood, the person's blood must contain HIV. Testing positive for HIV means that a person has HIV, but it does not necessarily mean that a person has AIDS.

HIV Transmission

There are certain ways HIV *can* and *cannot* be transmitted (**Figure 10.3.2**). HIV is found in blood, semen, vaginal fluids, and breast milk. HIV is *not* found in tears, saliva, or sweat.

HIV can be transmitted through sexual activity. It can also be transmitted if someone who has HIV gives birth to or breastfeeds a baby. HIV is *not* transmitted by mosquitoes or by kissing, spitting, shaking hands, sharing food, or using the same toilet seat.

HIV can also be transmitted through contaminated needles used for drugs or medications, tattoos, or body piercings. People who abuse drugs are more likely to share needles. This raises their risk of exposure to blood with HIV.

At one time, HIV was often transmitted in *blood transfusions*, or procedures in which people receive donated blood. In the United States, however, the blood supply is now screened for HIV, so transfusions are usually very safe.

Healthy, intact skin provides an effective barrier against HIV. HIV transmission is possible through open sores on skin, in the mouth, or on genitals. STIs cause inflammation, sores, and damage to skin. This breaks down barriers to HIV. Due to potential sores on skin, a person with STIs is also more at risk for HIV transmission.

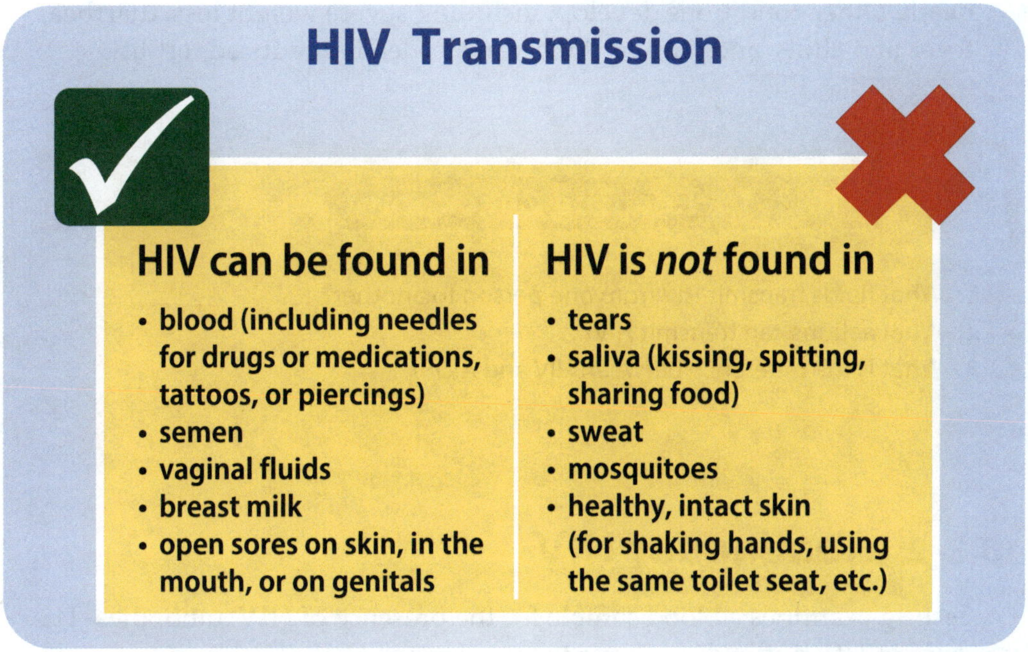

Figure 10.3.2 HIV can be transmitted in certain bodily fluids such as blood and semen, but not through other fluids such as saliva or sweat.

Can HIV be transmitted through shaking hands?

HIV Transmission

HIV can be found in
- blood (including needles for drugs or medications, tattoos, or piercings)
- semen
- vaginal fluids
- breast milk
- open sores on skin, in the mouth, or on genitals

HIV is *not* found in
- tears
- saliva (kissing, spitting, sharing food)
- sweat
- mosquitoes
- healthy, intact skin (for shaking hands, using the same toilet seat, etc.)

Goodheart-Willcox Publisher

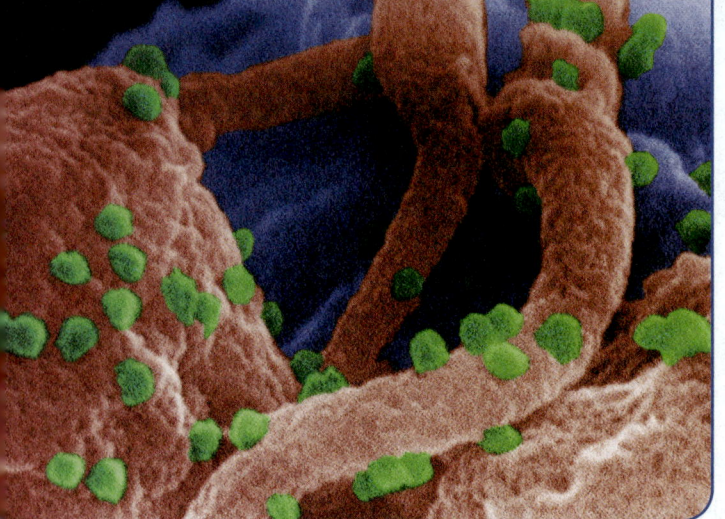

Courtesy of the Centers for Disease Control and Prevention

Figure 10.3.3 HIV (shown here in green) weakens the body's immune system by infecting and killing cells (shown in red).

Signs and Symptoms of HIV/AIDS

The signs and symptoms of HIV and AIDS depend on how far HIV has progressed. Without treatment, HIV progresses through three stages. The last stage of HIV is AIDS.

- **Stage 1: Acute HIV infection.** The first signs and symptoms of HIV may develop two to four weeks after HIV transmission. Some people develop no symptoms. Symptoms are often minor, and people may not know they are ill. Early symptoms can resemble a flu-like illness. People may develop fatigue and swollen, painful lymph nodes. Because of this, many people do not know they have been infected with HIV. However, the levels of virus in the blood are high during this stage (Figure 10.3.3). Acute HIV infections can result in reduced fertility.

- **Stage 2: Latency.** Stage 2 may cause no symptoms, and levels of HIV in the blood are low. This stage can last 10 or more years for some people. These people, called **long-term non-progressors**, pass through this stage very slowly. Others may progress through the stage more quickly. With treatment, this stage could last several decades or indefinitely. At the end of this stage, the immune system begins to work less effectively.

- **Stage 3: Acquired immunodeficiency syndrome (AIDS).** In AIDS, HIV has severely damaged the immune system. The body is attacked by unusual or normally harmless pathogens. These cause **opportunistic infections**, which take advantage of the body's weakened immune system and can result in death. Other conditions develop, including severe weight loss, diarrhea, fever and chills, and nausea. AIDS can also lead to reduced fertility.

10.3–1 Reading Checkpoint

1. What fluids transmit HIV from one person to another?
2. What actions can transmit HIV?
3. What is the difference between HIV and AIDS?

10.3–2 Testing for HIV

Testing examines a blood sample for the presence of HIV antibodies. The presence of HIV antibodies means the presence of HIV.

A person may not develop HIV antibodies until weeks or months after exposure to HIV. For example, if a person thinks they were exposed, but they get a negative blood test, HIV testing should be repeated after three more months have passed.

Test results are available in a few days. The rapid version of the test gives results in 20 minutes. HIV tests are often performed in doctors' offices and hospital labs. However, HIV tests may be done in clinics and other locations. HIV test sites can be found by searching the internet or by contacting the Centers for Disease Control and Prevention (CDC).

A home version of the HIV test is available without a prescription. The test is inexpensive, fast, painless, and private. If a person's home test shows the presence of HIV, they should see a doctor for a test to confirm the results.

HIV testing benefits both the individual and society. Sexually active people should be tested every year. They should also test every time they switch sexual partners. Testing allows people to begin treatment as soon as possible.

Treatment reduces the chance of developing AIDS. Testing also enables people to take steps to prevent transmission of HIV. For these reasons, testing is the key to controlling HIV transmission within society. Sadly, some people with HIV do not know they have it (Figure 10.3.4).

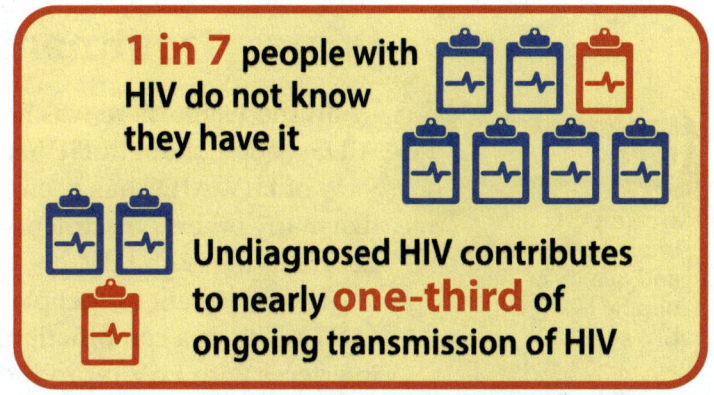

Figure 10.3.4 Sexually active people who have undiagnosed HIV can unknowingly transmit the virus to others.

How much of ongoing HIV transmission is due to undiagnosed HIV?

HIV Test Results Are Confidential and Private

The *Health Insurance Portability and Accountability Act (HIPAA)* is a federal law. Under this law, the results of a person's HIV test must be kept secret.

Healthcare workers must report positive test results to the state. This is because states track and study the number of HIV cases. The test results, however, are reported without identifying the individual.

People living with HIV are encouraged to share their results with sexual partners. By sharing their test results, people can protect their partners. Some cities and states have partner-notification laws. These laws require people living with HIV or their doctors to notify sexual or needle-sharing partners.

Protecting Individuals with HIV from Discrimination

Individuals living with HIV may face discrimination in society and in their workplaces. *Discrimination* is the unfair treatment of a certain group of people. For example, an employer might make assumptions about how many sick days a person with HIV might take. The federal government seeks to prevent this type of discrimination.

Two federal laws protect the rights of people with HIV. The *Americans with Disabilities Act (ADA) of 1990* and the *Rehabilitation Act of 1973* prohibit discrimination against people with HIV. This means that people with HIV cannot be denied jobs, benefits, education, services, or other rights because of their HIV status. These laws also protect the families of people living with HIV.

10.3-2 Reading Checkpoint

1. How often should a sexually active person be tested for HIV?
2. Where can a person go to be tested for HIV?

10.3-3 Treatment for HIV/AIDS

Essential Idea

Treatments improve the health and quality of life for people living with HIV/AIDS.

In the 1980s, there was no effective treatment for people living with HIV/AIDS. People thought HIV/AIDS was an untreatable, fatal disease. Today, this view of HIV/AIDS has been proven untrue. HIV is now a chronic condition like many others. Treatments have improved the health and quality of life for people living with HIV.

The treatment for people living with HIV is **antiretroviral therapy (ART).** This is a combination of medications, sometimes called a *cocktail*. ART interferes with HIV reproduction in the body. People should start ART as soon as possible after getting a positive HIV test.

The goal of ART is to reduce the amount of HIV in a person's blood. Today, ART can reduce the amount of HIV to the point that tests cannot even detect the virus. People using ART regularly also do not transmit HIV. Some people taking ART never develop AIDS.

10.3-3 Reading Checkpoint

1. What is the treatment for people living with HIV?
2. How does the treatment work?

10.3-4 HIV Prevention

Essential Idea

Sexual abstinence, using condoms, not sharing needles, and taking certain medications can help people avoid contracting HIV.

Understanding how HIV/AIDS is transmitted helps people avoid contracting HIV. In the United States, HIV is most often transmitted through sexual activity and needle sharing.

Methods of preventing other STIs also help prevent HIV (Figure 10.3.5). If you are taking a medication that needs to be injected, never share needles with another person. Always use a new, sterile needle for each injection. If you get a piercing or tattoo, make sure the piercer or tattoo artist is licensed. Be sure they use a new, sterile needle and new ink for each customer.

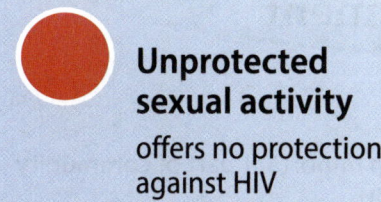 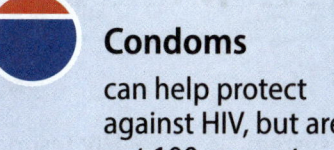 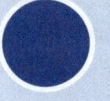

Unprotected sexual activity offers no protection against HIV

Condoms can help protect against HIV, but are not 100 percent effective

Abstinence is the only method 100 percent effective in preventing HIV transmission through sexual activity

Goodheart-Willcox Publisher

Figure 10.3.5 Many methods prevent STIs, but abstinence is the only method that is 100 percent effective. *What is the only method that is 100 percent effective in preventing HIV transmission from sexual activity?*

Certain medications can also reduce a person's risk of contracting HIV. These include PrEP and PEP (**Figure 10.3.6**).

- **Pre-exposure prophylaxis (PrEP)** is a type of ART intended for people who have a high risk of contracting HIV. PrEP reduces a person's risk of contracting HIV from sexual activity by more than 90 percent. When combined with other methods, PrEP reduces the risk to near zero. PrEP also reduces the risk of contracting HIV from shared needles by more than 70 percent. PrEP does not prevent other STIs.
- **Post-exposure prophylaxis (PEP)** is a type of ART a person can take within 72 hours of exposure to HIV to help prevent transmission. PEP is only intended for emergency use. For example, some healthcare workers can be exposed through a needle injury. Some people might be exposed from sexual activity, sexual assault, or from shared needles.

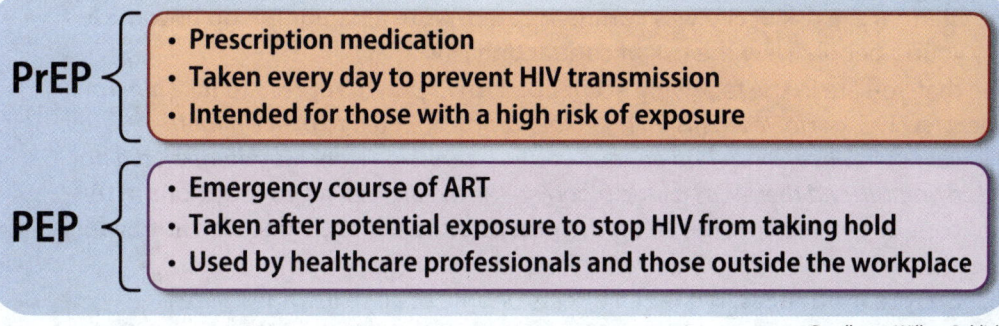

Figure 10.3.6 PrEP and PEP can help prevent HIV transmission.

Goodheart-Willcox Publisher

10.3–4 Reading Checkpoint

1. What are four ways to prevent HIV?
2. Explain what PrEP and PEP are and how they are used to prevent HIV.

Lesson 10.3 Review and Assessment

Reading Summary

10.3–1 HIV is a virus that weakens the immune system. HIV can progress into AIDS, a health condition in which the immune system cannot fight infections.

10.3–1 HIV is found in blood, semen, vaginal fluids, and breast milk. Activities that involve contact with these fluids, such as sexual activity and needle sharing, can transmit HIV.

10.3–2 Testing for the presence of HIV antibodies involves examining a sample of blood. HIV testing is an important part of community and public health.

10.3–3 Antiretroviral therapy (ART) is the main treatment for HIV/AIDS. With early treatment, a person living with HIV may never develop AIDS.

10.3–4 HIV prevention involves sexual abstinence, using a condom, not sharing needles, and taking medications that reduce transmission.

Critical Thinking

1. **Predict.** Do you think young people consider the risk of HIV when engaging in sexual activity? Defend your answer.
2. **Cause and effect.** What are the potential consequences, for the health of self and others, if someone engages in sexual activity and does not get regularly tested for HIV?

Develop Your Skills

1. **Analyze Influences.** Social media, TV shows, and songs often portray sexual activity with little to no consequences. Within small groups or as a class, brainstorm examples. Describe the message that is portrayed and determine whether the risk of HIV was communicated. Write a paragraph on how these messages impact the way young people view the risk of contracting HIV.
2. **Make Decisions.** Imagine that you are in the following scenario: *Carter's parents agreed to take him to get his ear pierced in the next few weeks. However, his friend's older brother offered to pierce it for free. Carter watched as two older boys went first. Since Carter had already gotten permission from his parents, it did not seem like a big deal. It looked painful, and there was a little blood on the needle.* List all your options in this scenario. List the pros and cons of each option. Based on the pros and cons, make a decision as to your best course of action.
3. **Access Information and Analyze Influences.** While HIV affects people of all sexes, ages, races, nationalities, and ethnic origins, some groups are more affected than others. Using valid and reliable sources, research how different groups of individuals are affected by HIV. Determine what factors influence the risk of HIV among groups. Write a summary or create a graphic organizer of your findings. Cite your valid sources.

Module 11 Sexual Health

- **Lesson 11.1** What Is Sexuality?
- **Lesson 11.2** Sexual Feelings and Abstinence
- **Lesson 11.3** Pregnancy Prevention

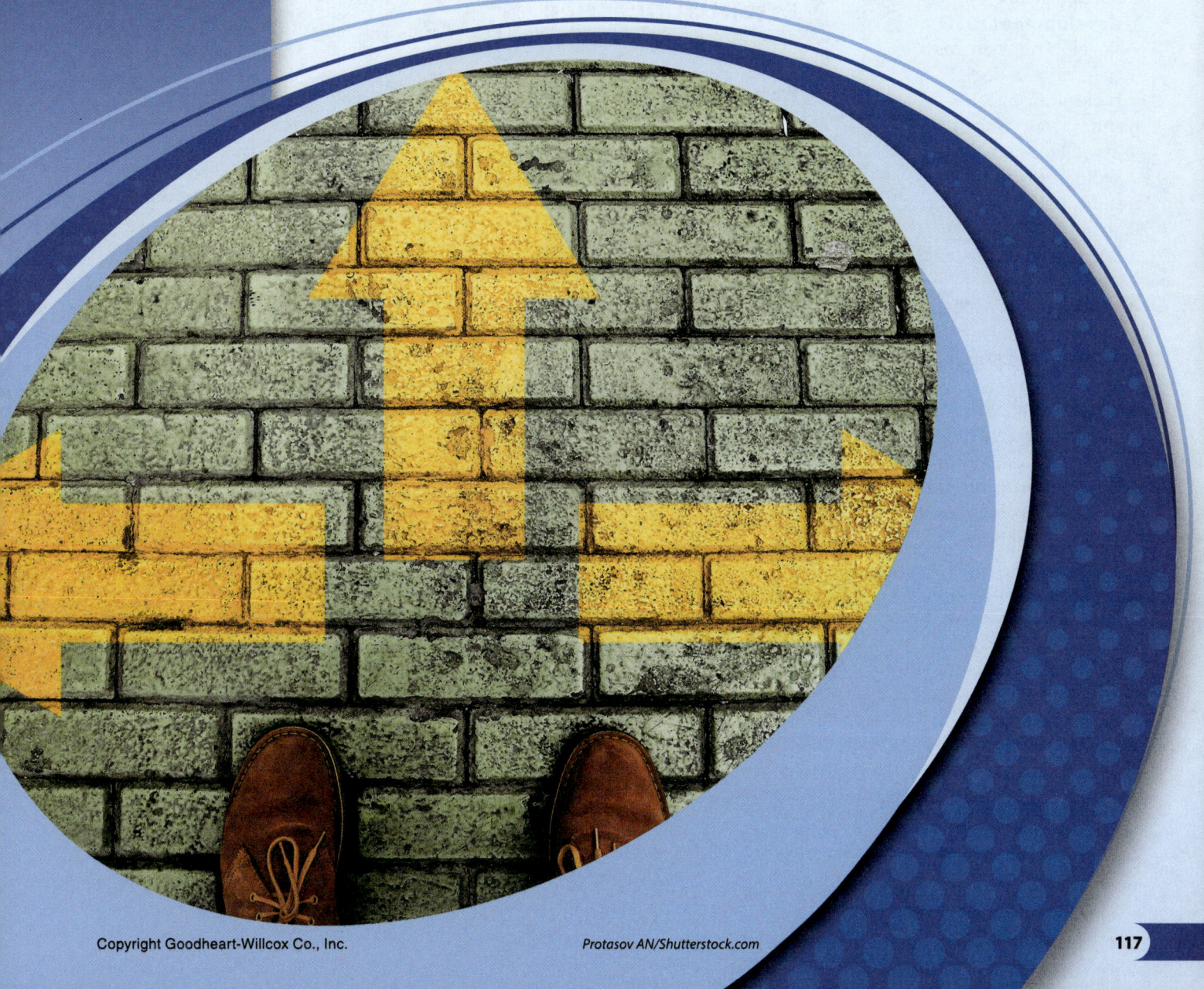

Lesson 11.1 What Is Sexuality?

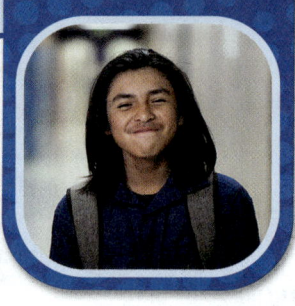

Key Terms

sexuality a person's biological sex, sexual feelings, sexual orientation, gender identity, and gender expression

biological sex individual's sex, male or female, as determined by their sex chromosomes, genes, hormones, and reproductive organs

disorder of sex development (DSD) development process of having an unclear biological sex

gender traits a society associates with a particular biological sex

gender roles behaviors society considers "appropriate" for a certain gender

gender identity deeply held thoughts and feelings a person has about their gender

transgender having a gender identity different from one's biological sex

sexual orientation lasting pattern of romantic and sexual attraction

homophobia hostility, anger, exclusion, and violence directed at LGBTQ+ individuals

transphobia discrimination and violence directed at people who are transgender

Learning Outcomes

Look for the skills icon  to practice health skills.
After studying this lesson, you will be able to
- 11.1–1 **Explain** the concept of biological sex.
- 11.1–2 **Describe** gender roles, gender identity, and gender expression.
- 11.1–3 **Identify** various sexual orientations.
- 11.1–4 **Understand** the challenges associated with discrimination and violence.

Essential Question

What are the parts of a person's sexuality?

Reading and Notetaking Activity

On a separate sheet of paper, draw four boxes labeled for each of the sections in this lesson. As you read this lesson, organize your notes in the appropriate boxes.

Biological Sex
- Determined by sex chromosomes, genes, hormones, and reproductive organs.
-

Gender, Gender Identity, and Gender Expression
-
-

Sexual Orientation
-
-

Challenges in the LGBTQ+ Community
-
-

Goodheart-Willcox Publisher

Lesson image:
THEPALMER/E+ via Getty Images

Introduction

This year is not the first time Carter has heard the word *sexuality*. Still, he does not understand how the word applies to him. Last year, Carter's older sister told him that she is attracted to girls. Now, Carter's friend Alia told him she is not sure about her gender identity.

Carter does not feel attracted to anyone at school yet. He wonders what it will feel like when he is attracted to someone. He questions whether he has sexuality, since he does not want to have sex.

Sexuality is a part of human life. A person's sexuality is a part of their identity. You do not have to be sexually active or even interested in sex to learn about your sexuality. Sexuality is about more than your sexual anatomy, chromosomes, or body parts. Parts of **sexuality** include a person's biological sex, sexual feelings, sexual orientation, gender identity, and gender expression (**Figure 11.1.1**).

Sexuality involves how a person looks, feels, thinks, and acts. It affects how other people view and treat a person. It influences what roles the person plays in family and society.

Young people may have questions about sexuality. For medically accurate information, young people can speak to a doctor or a school nurse. It is also important for young people to talk to their parent, guardian, or other trusted adult.

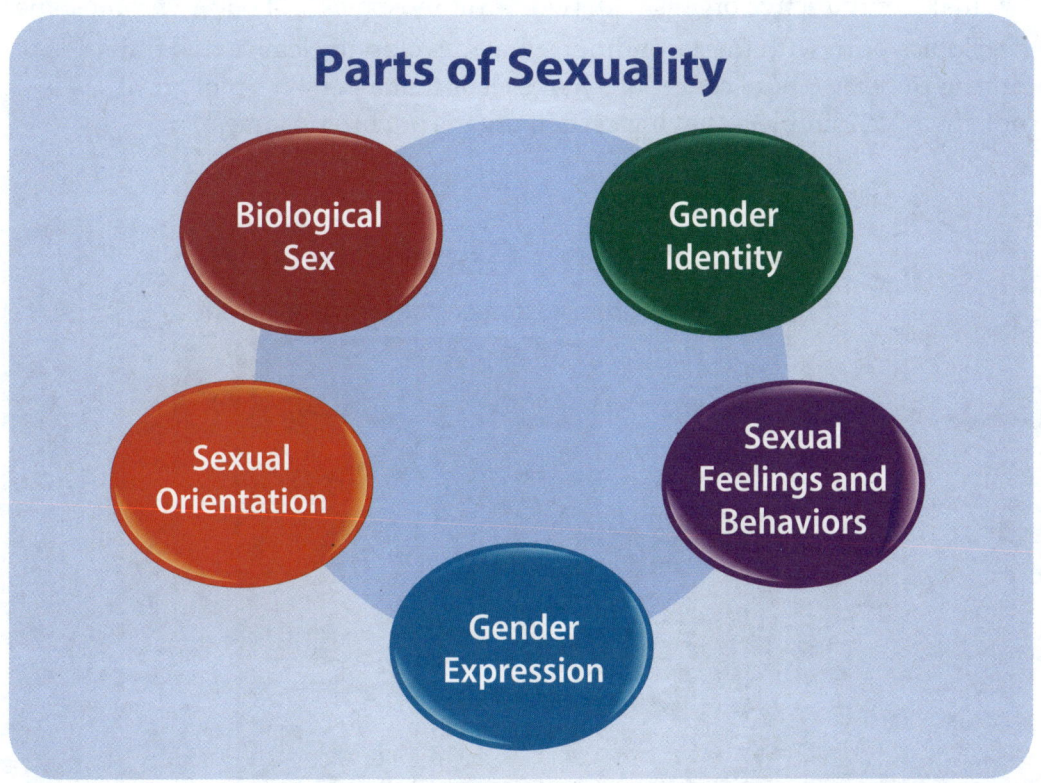

Figure 11.1.1
Sexuality is part of a person's identity. There are five main parts to a person's sexuality.

Goodheart-Willcox Publisher

Lesson   What Is Sexuality?

11.1-1 Biological Sex

Essential Idea

A person's biological sex, whether an individual is male or female, is determined by sex chromosomes, genes, hormones, and reproductive organs.

Biological sex is whether an individual is genetically and physically a male or female. It is determined by two sex chromosomes, called X and Y chromosomes. One sex chromosome is inherited from each biological parent. People who are genetically male typically have one X and one Y chromosome. People who are genetically female typically have two X chromosomes (**Figure 11.1.2**). Sex chromosomes help direct the development of the reproductive organs and other sexual traits.

By the seventh week of prenatal development, a fetus' sex chromosomes can usually be determined by a doctor through a blood test. After the eighteenth week, the external reproductive organs of a fetus can be seen using ultrasound.

At birth, babies are often assigned a biological sex based on the appearance of their external reproductive organs. However, as many as 1–2 percent of live births result in babies born with an unclear biological sex. This development process is called a **disorder of sex development (DSD)**. Some people who have an unclear biological sex prefer to identify as *intersex*.

In most cases, this difference in development happens because reproductive organs have not developed fully. In other cases, external reproductive organs may not match the baby's sex chromosomes. Babies can be born with the following conditions:

- female reproductive organs and XY chromosomes
- male reproductive organs and XX chromosomes
- female reproductive organs with only one X chromosome
- male reproductive organs with two X chromosomes and one Y chromosome

Babies born with these conditions may develop unclear sexual traits during puberty. These conditions make clear that a person's biological sex is not always as simple as having certain organs or chromosomes.

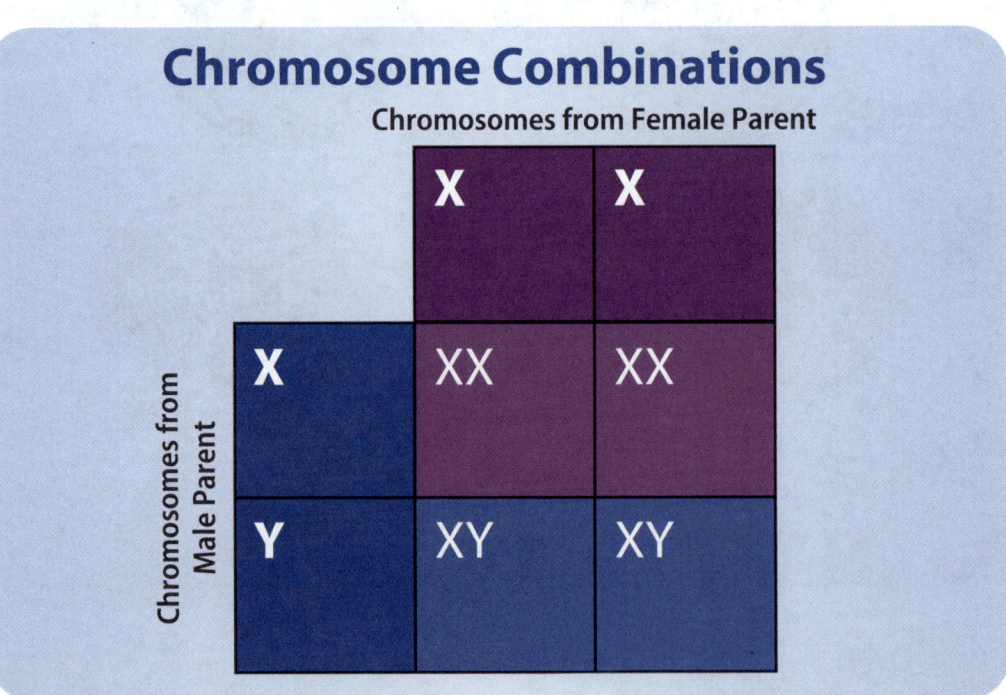

Figure 11.1.2 People who are genetically female typically have the chromosome combination XX. People who are genetically male typically have the chromosome combination XY.

Which sex chromosome is typically present only in the male parent?

Goodheart-Willcox Publisher

11.1–1 Reading Checkpoint

1. How do sex chromosomes differ between people who are genetically male and female?
2. Provide two examples of why it might not be simple to assign a baby's biological sex at birth.

11.1-2 Gender, Gender Identity, and Gender Expression

Gender is the behaviors and traits a society associates with a person's biological sex. Expectations of how people fit into genders vary between cultures and societies. Gender identity and gender expression also have to do with the concept of gender.

Gender Expectations

Views of gender vary among societies and cultures. These views also change over time. So do gender roles. **Gender roles** are behaviors a society considers "appropriate" for a gender.

In the United States, gender is often viewed as *masculine* or *feminine*. The traits people think are masculine and feminine are typically complete opposites. For example, this view may expect men to be aggressive and women to be passive. This is an example of the *gender binary*, or the idea that the genders of man and woman are entirely opposite.

This is not how people really behave. People do not have only masculine or feminine traits. Most people's behavior lies in between the two extremes (**Figure 11.1.3**). For example, a boy can be a competitive athlete and still take care of a younger sibling. A girl can be a loving friend and still be dedicated to pursuing a career as a computer programmer.

The gender binary and social factors can make young people feel insecure about gender. Some young people feel unsure of how others see them. Their friends and family may hold gender stereotypes that pressure them to act a certain way.

Gender stereotypes are fixed views, roles, and traits people associate with a gender. However, many people do not fit these gender roles.

Gender Identity

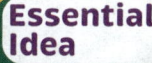

Essential Idea

Gender identity is a person's deeply held feeling about their gender. Gender expression is how a person outwardly displays gender.

Gender identity is your deeply held thoughts and feelings about your gender. Children learn their gender identity early in life. In fact, most three-year-olds easily identify their gender. A child's sense of their gender becomes well-established around five years of age (**Figure 11.1.4**).

Some people identify with the gender identity associated with their biological sex. These people are called *cisgender*. Some people may realize they

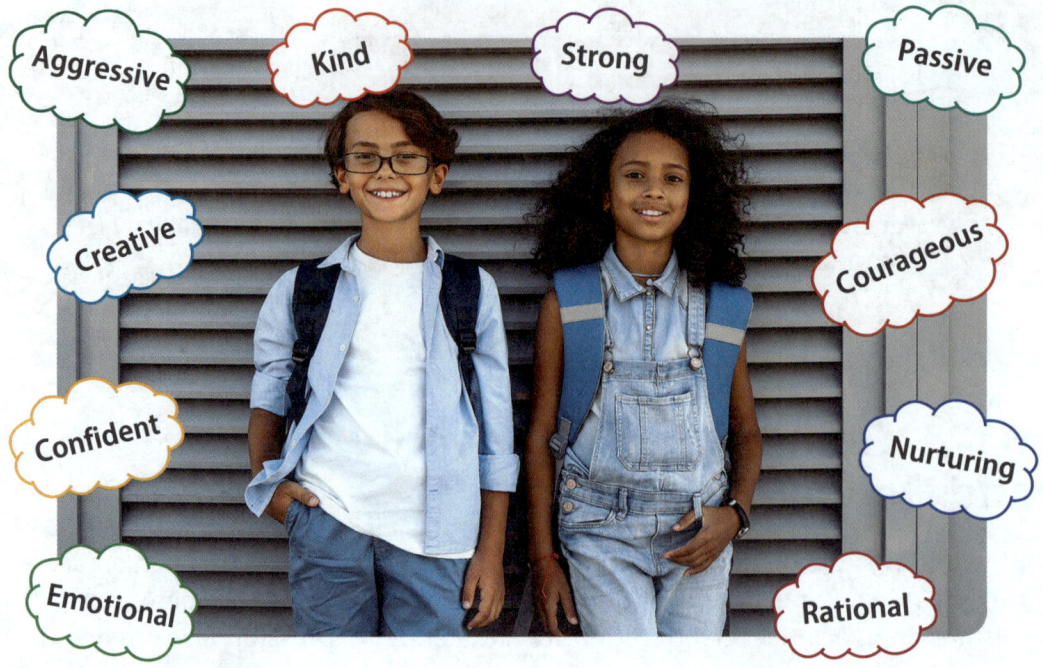

Figure 11.1.3 No one is only masculine or only feminine. Most people have both masculine and feminine traits.

Inside Creative House/Shutterstock.com

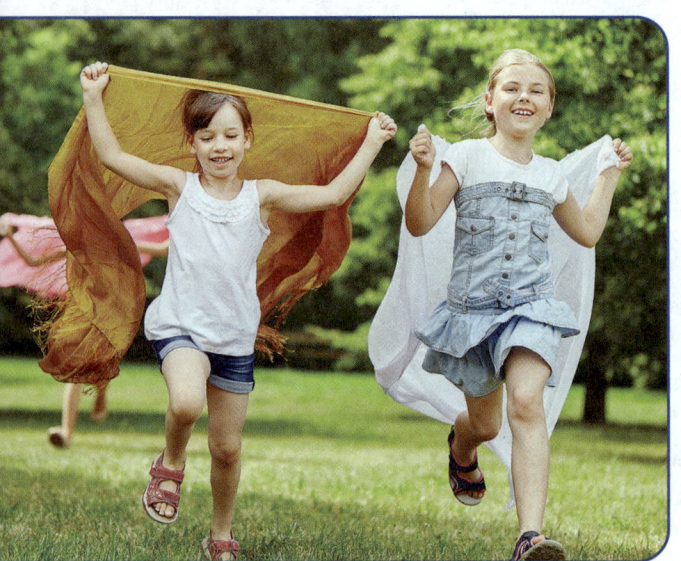

Robert Kneschke/Shutterstock.com

Figure 11.1.4 During childhood, most boys play with other boys, and girls play with other girls. This may support a child's sense of gender identity. It is also normal, however, for some children to role-play other genders or play with children of a different gender.

do not identify with the gender identity assigned to them. This happens for many reasons.

When people are *gender nonconforming*, their appearance and behaviors do not align with the gender associated with their biological sex. A person with a gender identity different from their biological sex is **transgender**. For example, a person may be born with female sexual anatomy but identify as a boy. Someone who is born with male sexual anatomy may identify as neither a man or a woman.

Some people view themselves as *nonbinary*. This means their gender identity may fall outside of the categories of man or woman. For example, people may identify with no gender (*agender*) or two genders (*bigender*). Some people may have a *fluid*, or changing, gender identity.

Many social factors affect the relationship a person has with gender identity. Pressures can come from a person's friends and peers. Family and culture also impact a person's view of gender identity. As a result, some people who are transgender may be confused about their gender identity for many years.

Some people prefer to use pronouns that match their gender identity. For example, a person who identifies as a woman might ask others to use *she/her* when speaking about her. A person identifying as a man might prefer to use *he/him*. Sometimes a person chooses to use nongendered pronouns such as *they/them*. Using people's preferred pronouns is a way of respecting their identity.

Breaking the Myth of Gendered Personality Traits

Personality traits are often described as either "masculine" or "feminine."

Example: aggressive or empathetic

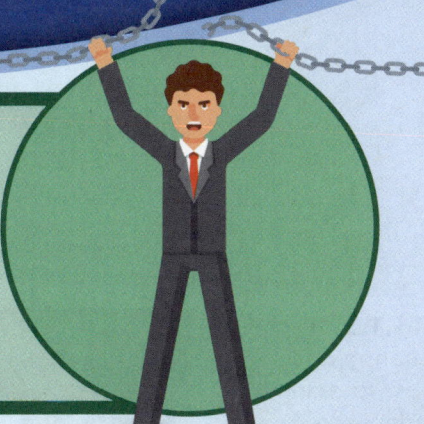

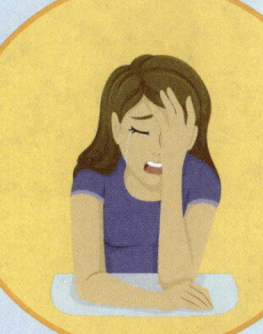
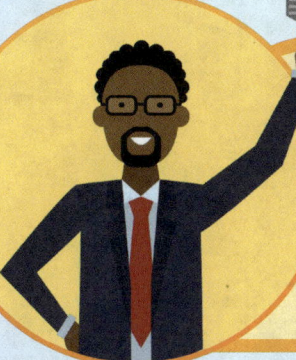

These gendered traits tend to be polar opposites.

Example: emotional versus rational

No one is fully one extreme or the other, and the traits you have are not determined by your biological sex.

Example: courageous or powerful

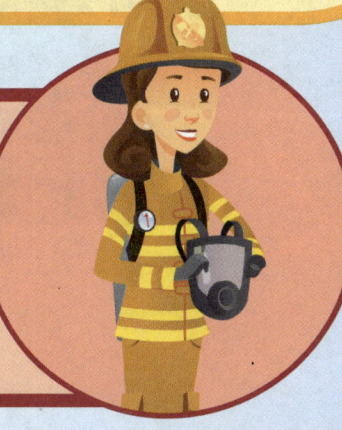

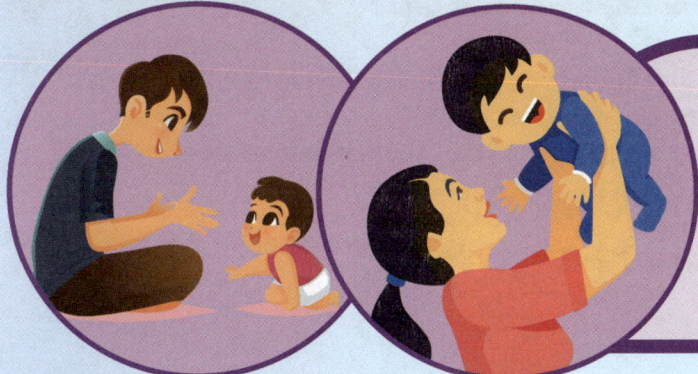

Everyone has the potential, as a person, to develop each of these personality traits.

Example: parental and nurturing

Top to bottom: Iconic Bestiary/Shutterstock.com; Lorelyn Medina/Shutterstock.com; Inspiring/Shutterstock.com; Serenkly/Shutterstock.com; Iconic Bestiary/Shutterstock.com; ziiinvn/Shutterstock.com

Gender Expression

Gender expression is the way you outwardly display gender. This could include the clothes you wear, your physical appearance, and your behaviors.

Some people feel comfortable expressing their gender identity through their appearance and behaviors. Other people, however, may not feel comfortable or safe expressing their gender identity. People may choose to change their appearance, clothing, and name to match their gender identity (**Figure 11.1.5**).

Figure 11.1.5 People who are transgender may choose to change their gender expression to match their gender identity.

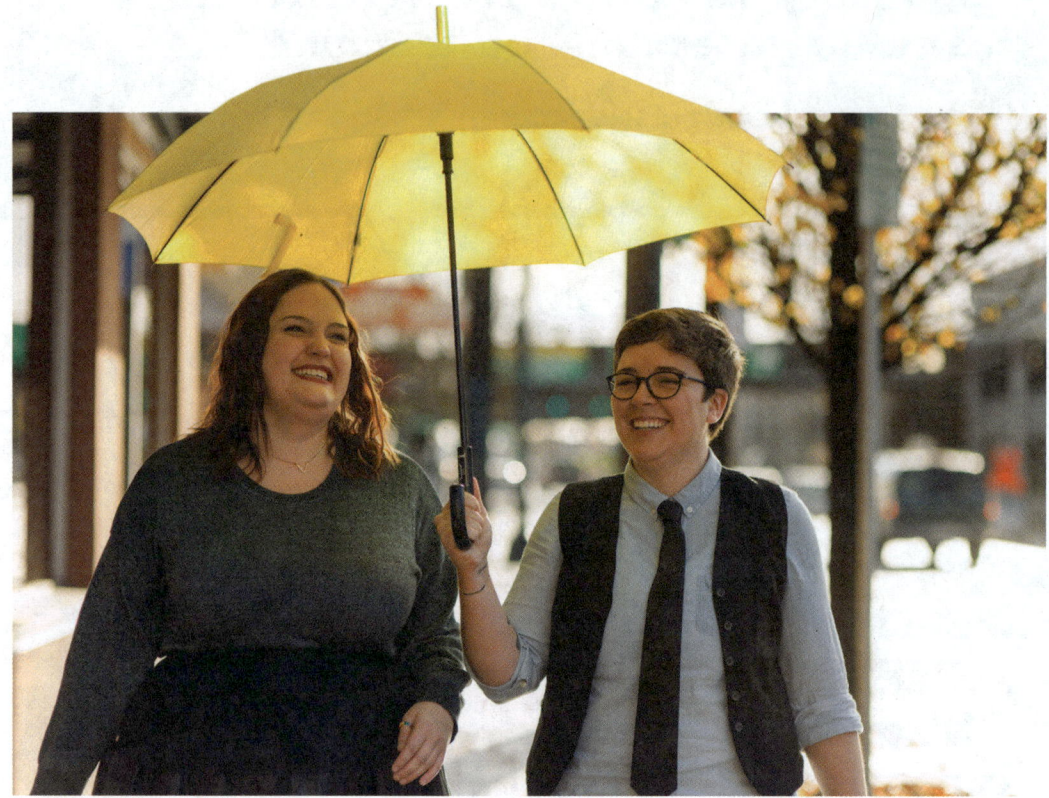

iStock.com/FatCamera

11.1–2 Reading Checkpoint

1. How are gender, gender identity, and gender expression related? Provide an example of each in your explanation.
2. What connections can you make between the information presented and the real world?

11.1-3 Sexual Orientation

Sexual orientation is the lasting pattern of a person's romantic and/or sexual attraction to other people. Various terms are used to describe sexual orientation. People may or may not identify themselves using these terms (**Figure 11.1.6**).

Not all young people develop these feelings at the same time. People develop at different rates. Some know their sexual orientation early in puberty. Some people may know earlier in childhood, and some later. Social factors affect people's views of sexual orientation. These factors include peers, family, society, culture, and the media they consume.

All orientations can be found in people of all races, ethnicities, cultures, countries, and social and economic backgrounds. Many factors, including a person's genes, environment, and experiences, influence a person's sexual orientation. Some factors are unknown.

> **Essential Idea**
>
> Sexual orientation is a person's pattern of attraction to other people.

Heterosexual or straight
For men, being sexually attracted to women. For women, being sexually attracted to men.

Gay or lesbian
Being sexually attracted to someone of the same gender.

Bisexual
Being sexually attracted to someone of the same gender and other genders.

Asexual
Not having sexual attraction to anyone.

Figure 11.1.6 These are just a few examples of terms people may use to describe their sexual orientation.

> Which term is used to describe not having sexual attraction to anyone?

Scalia Media/Shutterstock.com

11.1-3 Reading Checkpoint

1. What are two examples of terms people may use to describe a sexual orientation? State the terms and their definitions.
2. When might a person come to understand their sexual orientation? Explain.

11.1-4 Challenges in the LGBTQ+ Community

LGBTQ+ stands for *lesbian*, *gay*, *bisexual*, *transgender*, and *queer or questioning*. The plus sign is used to include people with other sexual orientations and gender identities. The acronym *LGBTQ* is sometimes expanded to include *I* (intersex) and *A* (asexual). Some people are active in trying to make sure LGBTQ+ people are treated fairly and have the same basic rights as all people.

Questions About Sexuality

It is normal for young people to have questions or feel confused about their sexuality. At times, some young people who are heterosexual may feel attracted to the same gender. This does not mean they must be gay, lesbian, or bisexual. For example, a girl might develop a crush on another girl or female celebrity. This fairly common feeling is related to increased hormone levels in puberty. In time, most people develop a clearer sense of their sexual orientation.

Like other young people, those who are LGBTQ+ may want to discuss their romantic feelings, dating, and sexuality. However, they may feel they need to hide this part of themselves.

From a young age, people who are LGBTQ+ may feel out of place. They may even feel rejected by others (**Figure 11.1.7**).

If you want to learn more about sexual orientation, turn to valid and reliable sources. Ask your parent or guardian, the school nurse, a doctor, a counselor, or a therapist. Visit websites provided by government agencies or experts in the field.

Discrimination and Violence

People who are LGBTQ+ sometimes face unfair treatment. They may have to deal with other people's negative attitudes and actions, sometimes daily. For example, in recent years, nearly 25 percent of young people who are LGBTQ+ were bullied in person at school. Almost 30 percent were electronically bullied. The negative attitudes may even come from the family members of the person who is LGBTQ+.

The term **homophobia** refers to hostility, anger, exclusion, and violence directed at people who are LGBTQ+. **Transphobia** is discrimination and violence directed at people who are transgender.

These attitudes can harm the health of people who are LGBTQ+. Young people who are LGBTQ+ are at a greater risk for depression and anxiety. They

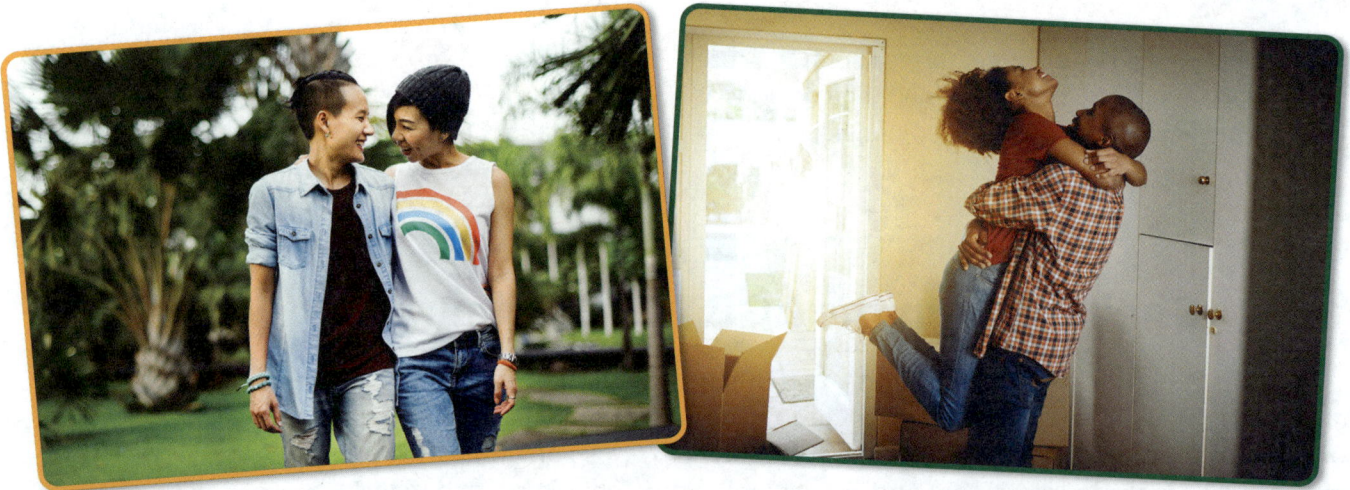

Left to right: iStock.com/Rawpixel; iStock.com/Peopleimages

Figure 11.1.7 People, no matter their sexual orientation or gender identity, are unique individuals. Each person may dress and behave in different ways from others of the same orientation or identity.

are also at a higher risk of dropping out of school and running away from home.

To avoid harassment, some people who are LGBTQ+ hide their sexual orientation or gender identity. However, it can be difficult and painful to deny this basic part of who they are.

Good support systems can help people who are LGBTQ+ feel safe. Social support can also help them feel at ease with themselves. Many feel relieved when they tell trusted people about their sexual orientation or gender identity.

BUILDING YOUR SKILLS — Community Connections

Promoting Acceptance, Tolerance, and Unity

Has anyone ever teased or treated you badly because of your biological sex, gender identity, or sexual orientation? Have you ever witnessed people being treated this way?

If so, you probably know how negative words and actions can hurt a person's self-esteem and confidence. Discrimination and harassment of any kind are wrong. It is important to stand up and use your voice to speak out against violence in any form.

Schools around the world have taken steps to discourage discrimination and harassment. Many have created student clubs or safe zones for young people. The goal of these is to promote acceptance, tolerance, and unity among people of all sexualities. Even if you are not part of a student club, you play a part in encouraging unity and tolerance. Owning this part and speaking up can help people of all sexualities feel accepted.

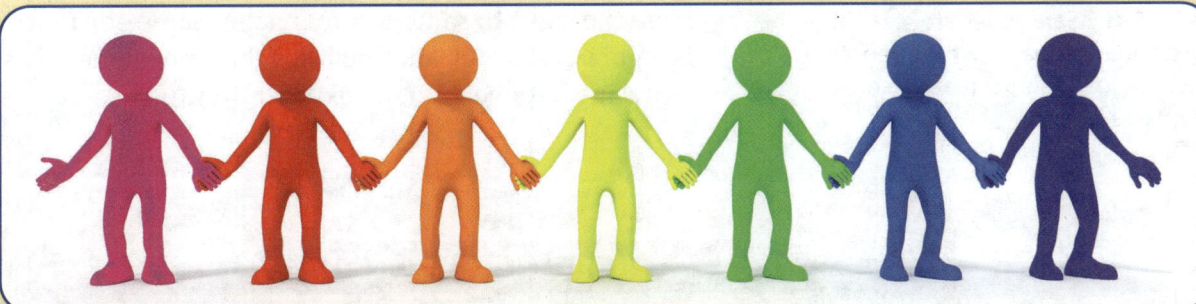

Markus Gann/Shutterstock.com

Practice Your Skills — Advocate for Health

Assess how well your school promotes acceptance, tolerance, and unity among people of all sexualities. It includes how students are treated by school staff and other students. Use the following steps to improve your school climate:

1. In small groups, discuss ways to improve the school climate for all students to feel accepted, regardless of sexual orientation or gender identity. One student in the group should take notes about these suggestions.
2. As a class, share these suggestions. Choose three to five suggestions that are realistic for your school.
3. Share your class suggestions with a student club that promotes acceptance, tolerance, and unity. If a club like this or a safe zone does not exist at your school, consider creating one. Work with the club to carry out the suggestions.

Support for Young People Who Are LGBTQ+

Having an accepting group of people around them can help young people who are LGBTQ+ deal with daily challenges. Many schools have created student clubs, as well as safe zones, for students who are LGBTQ+ and those who support them (**Figure 11.1.8**).

An *ally* in the LGBTQ+ community is a person who supports the rights and safety of other people who are LGTBQ+. Anyone can be an ally of the LGBTQ+ community. LGBTQ+ allies include many people who are heterosexual or cisgender.

Federal laws help protect people who are LGBTQ+ from discrimination and violence.

- The *Civil Service Reform Act of 1978* and *Civil Rights Act of 1991* prohibit employers from discriminating against workers based on their sexual orientation.
- Title IX of the *Education Amendments of 1972* prohibits education programs that receive federal money from discriminating based on a person's sex. This includes biological sex, sexual orientation, and gender identity.
- The *Matthew Shepard and James Byrd, Jr. Hate Crimes Prevention Act* protects people from crimes based on a person's sexual orientation and race.
- In 2015, the United States Supreme Court decided people have the right to same-sex marriage. Same-sex marriage is legal in all states and includes the same benefits as marriage between heterosexual individuals.

Safe Zones...
- help people in the LGBTQ+ community feel welcomed.
- are spaces where students know they will be accepted.
- increase inclusiveness and support.
- lead to greater feelings of safety, tolerance, and respect for students who are LGBTQ+ as well as the community.

Goodheart-Willcox Publisher

Figure 11.1.8 Safe zones are parts of a school created as spaces where people in the LGBTQ+ community feel welcomed and accepted.

11.1–4 Reading Checkpoint

1. What are some challenges that individuals in the LGBTQ+ community face?
2. How can an individual and a community support young people who are LGBTQ+?

Lesson 11.1 Review and Assessment

Reading Summary

11.1–1 Biological sex is determined by sex chromosomes (XX or XY). Some babies are born with a disorder of sex development (DSD). People with this difference in development may identify as intersex.

11.1–2 A person's deeply held thoughts and feelings about gender is gender identity. Gender expression is the way a person outwardly displays gender.

11.1–3 Sexual orientation is the lasting pattern of romantic and sexual attraction. Examples of sexual orientations include heterosexual, gay, lesbian, bisexual, and asexual.

11.1–4 LGBTQ+ stands for lesbian, gay, bisexual, transgender, and queer or questioning. People who are LGBTQ+ sometimes face unfair treatment and violence. Laws help protect people from this discrimination and violence.

Critical Thinking

1. **Analyze.** How do the media, family, peers, and culture shape expectations for gender in society? How do these expectations influence gender expression?
2. **Interpret.** Why might it be challenging for young people to accept others with sexualities different from themselves? How can people overcome these challenges?

Develop Your Skills

1. **Advocate for Health.** With a partner, choose one topic related to sexuality that was discussed in this lesson. Educate others about your chosen topic. Create a poster, flyer, social media post, or other creative product about your topic. In your product, include a slogan about acceptance and information on your chosen topic. Also include a valid community resource that can provide support on sexuality. Be prepared to share your message with the class.
2. **Access Information.** Research websites and local resources that provide information about sexuality. Choose one local resource or website to present to the class. Create a digital presentation about your resource and explain why you do or do not consider it a valid source and if you would recommend it to your peers. Then, present this information in small groups or to the class.
3. **Make Decisions.** Imagine that you are in the following scenario: *At recess, one of your friends makes a rude comment about a student at school who is transgender. While you disagree with your friend's point of view, you feel the comment is harmless. The conversation continues until another classmate dares your friend to pull down the pants of the student who is transgender after the next class. Shocked, you are speechless.* With a partner, list your options in this situation. Explore the pros and cons of each option. Then, based on the pros and cons, decide your best course of action to protect the student who is transgender.

Lesson 11.2 Sexual Feelings and Abstinence

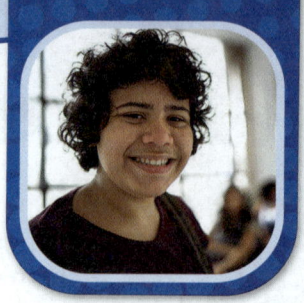

Key Terms

erection state in which the penis lengthens and hardens
arousal sexual excitement
wet dreams ejaculations that occur during sleep starting in male puberty
masturbation self-stimulation of the reproductive organ
sexual activity contact that stimulates the external reproductive organs, such as the penis or vagina

Learning Outcomes

Look for the skills icon  to practice health skills.
After studying this lesson, you will be able to
11.2–1 **Identify** the sexual changes that occur in puberty.
11.2–2 **Describe** the impacts of sexual activity.
11.2–3 **Explain** the benefits of abstinence and strategies that can support abstinence.

Essential Question

What sexual feelings may develop during puberty?

Reading and Notetaking Activity

As you read this lesson, take notes on Puberty, Sexual Activity, and Abstinence in a graphic organizer. At the bottom of each section, write the two most important facts you learned.

Puberty	Sexual Activity	Abstinence
• Notes:	• Notes:	• Notes:

• Important facts
  • 1:
  • 2:
	• Important facts
	  • 1:
	  • 2:
		• Important facts
		  • 1:
		  • 2:

Goodheart-Willcox Publisher

Lesson image:
FG Trade/E+ via Getty Images

Introduction

This year, Isabella confided in her friend Jimmy that she feels sexually attracted to one of their friends. Jimmy thinks that Isabella's feelings are probably normal. He wonders if it is also normal that he is not sexually attracted to anyone yet. It is not something that Jimmy and his friends have talked about. He knows that sexual relationships carry risks that young people can find difficult to handle.

11.2-1 Sexual Changes in Puberty

Puberty is the stage in which the body reaches sexual maturity. During puberty, hormones change a child's body into that of an adult (**Figure 11.2.1**). Over time, these hormones also cause new sexual feelings and emotions.

The Importance of Reproductive Hormones

Hormones are chemical messengers made by glands and released into the blood. Each type of hormone affects specific body parts.

The testes make *testosterone*, the male reproductive hormone. This hormone causes the testes, penis, and other male sexual traits to grow and develop. The ovaries produce the female reproductive hormone, *estrogen*. This hormone causes the ovaries, breasts, and other female sexual traits to grow and develop.

Physical Changes

During puberty, people develop mature sexual characteristics. *Primary sexual characteristics* refer to the reproductive organs. In male reproductive

Essential Idea

Puberty may bring new sexual feelings and emotions, such as arousal and curiosity about sexual activity.

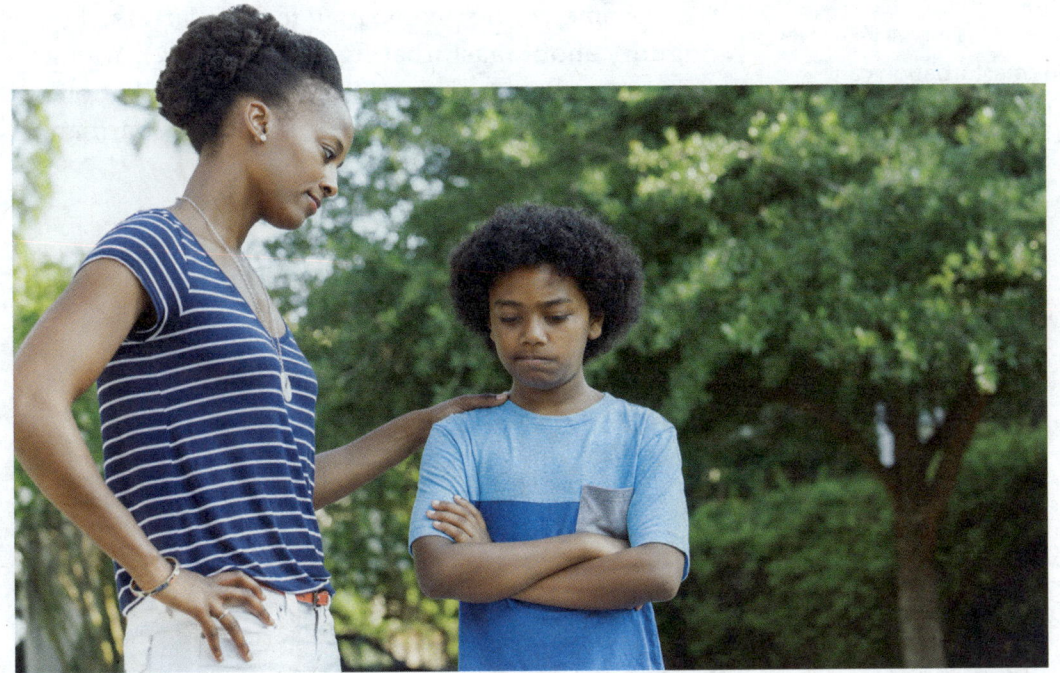

Figure 11.2.1 During puberty, young people grow quickly. Some may feel embarrassed about growing faster or slower than most of their friends and peers. It is normal for each person to grow at different rates.

iStock.com/kali9

Lesson Sexual Feelings and Abstinence

systems, the testes and penis mature and grow. In female reproductive systems, the ovaries, vagina, and labia mature and grow.

Secondary sexual characteristics are other traits of the mature body. People in male puberty may begin to have **erections**, in which the penis lengthens and hardens. Erections can occur in response to sexual excitement or for no reason at all.

Bodies change during female puberty, too. *Menstruation*, or the monthly shedding of blood and some tissues from the uterus, means that a female's body is releasing *eggs*, or female sex cells. Vaginal secretions also increase.

Early Sexual Feelings

Higher hormone levels can cause young people to feel sexually attracted to others. These new feelings may cause young people to ask themselves questions such as, "Am I normal?" and "Should I feel this way?" Like the physical changes of puberty, it is normal to experience these new sexual feelings. It is also normal to have not yet developed these sexual feelings.

Physical and emotional changes eventually lead to curiosity about sex. Sexual excitement, or **arousal**, is normal. Arousal can be caused by sexual thoughts, daydreams, or images. Young people may develop crushes on celebrities or people they know. Young people in male puberty may also experience erections and **wet dreams**, or ejaculations that occur during sleep.

During puberty, people might begin masturbating in response to sexual arousal. **Masturbation** is the self-stimulation of the reproductive organs. Masturbation is a sexual activity that allows people to safely release sexual tension.

Some young people may feel embarrassed or guilty about masturbating (Figure 11.2.2). Young people who have questions about masturbation can talk with a doctor, nurse, parent or guardian, or other trusted adult.

Goodheart-Willcox Publisher

Figure 11.2.2 Myths about masturbation can make young people feel embarrassed or guilty about masturbating. It is important to know the facts about masturbation.

11.2–1 Reading Checkpoint

1. What changes happen to the body due to reproductive hormones during puberty?
2. What questions do you think a middle school student might commonly have about puberty?

11.2-2 Sexual Activity

During puberty, some young people develop feelings of physical attraction to others. You may already notice these feelings or you may as your body develops. Feelings of romantic and physical attraction can feel new and intense. It is a normal part of how people develop during puberty.

Some young people may feel curious about sexual activities. **Sexual activity** is contact that stimulates the external reproductive organs, such as the penis or vagina. Engaging in any sexual activity has serious impacts that young people should carefully consider.

Even if young people do not engage in sexual activity, as they develop, they may want to talk about sex or make sexual comments. Some young people may be tempted to *sext*, or send sexual content such as text, photos, or videos. Sexting can have various negative impacts (**Figure 11.2.3**).

> **Essential Idea**
> Some young people may develop physical attraction to others and curiosity about sexual activities, including sexting.

Physical Impacts

Sexual activity can have many long-lasting physical impacts. For example, having vaginal sexual intercourse even once, and even for the first time, can lead to pregnancy and the birth of a baby (**Figure 11.2.4**). Because a young person's body is still developing, pregnancy comes with increased health risks to the pregnant person and baby.

Sexual activity can also lead to sexually transmitted infections (STIs). Some STIs do not show symptoms. This means some people do not know they have an STI. Even without symptoms, some STIs can lead to *infertility*, or a difficulty becoming pregnant. They can also cause genital warts, cervical cancer, or penile cancer. While some STIs are easily treated, others can affect a person for the rest of their life.

Emotional and Social Impacts

Hormones influence a person's emotions and behavior during and after sexual activity. They can cause feelings of bonding, closeness, and nurturing. These feelings can be very intense. They may be difficult for young people to manage. Young people may feel overwhelmed by these intense emotions

Impacts of Sexting

Legal
Sexting can be seen as harassment or child pornography and lead to jail time and fines.

Professional
Sexual photos that have been posted on the internet can negatively affect your future.

Social
Sharing sexts can lead to embarrassment, emotional distress, social isolation, poor body image, low self-esteem, depression, and anxiety.

notbad/Shutterstock.com

Figure 11.2.3 Sexting has negative impacts. If someone sends you a sext, delete the sext right away and tell a parent or other trusted adult.

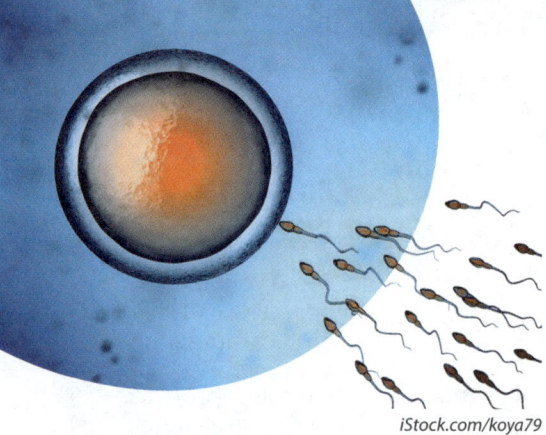

iStock.com/koya79

Figure 11.2.4 Fertilization occurs when a sperm enters an egg. Fertilization can result in pregnancy if the fertilized egg implants in the female's uterus.

because they are still learning the skills they need to form and maintain healthy dating relationships.

The intense feelings from sexual activity can make it difficult for young people to focus on individual growth and personal goals. It may also be difficult for a young person to build and maintain other relationships in addition to a sexual relationship.

With sexual activity, young people may also have to manage the stress of a possible pregnancy or STI. Dating relationships can be fun and rewarding without sexual activity.

BUILDING YOUR SKILLS — Digital Connections

The Impact of Sexting

Sexting refers to the sending and receiving of sexual content such as text, photos, or videos through electronic means. Sexting can be seen as harassment or child pornography and can result in serious legal impacts. Depending on the state that you live in, the impact of sexting can vary from an education program to a misdemeanor or a felony.

How you participate in the sexting also helps determine the size of the impact. You may not have control over what sexts you receive, but you do have control over how you respond to them and whether you share these sexts with other people. You also have control over whether you send sexts to others.

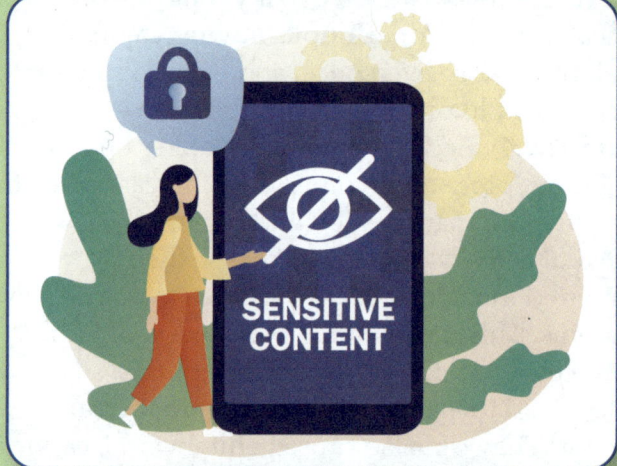

Marta Sher/Shutterstock.com

 Practice Your Skills — Access Information

How much do you know about your state laws regarding sexting? Research a valid and reliable source of information to learn more about the legal impact of sexting in your state. Gather the following information on sexting among minors:

- Is sexting among minors illegal in your state?
- In your state, what is the legal impact of sending a sext to another minor?
- In your state, is it a crime to receive a sext from another minor? What is the legal impact?

Compare your findings with a partner. Be prepared to participate in a student-led discussion and ask additional questions.

11.2–2 Reading Checkpoint

1. What are the potential negative impacts of sexting?
2. What are the physical, emotional, and social impacts of engaging in sexual activity?

11.2-3 Abstinence

Many young people recognize the potential impacts of early sexual activity and decide to choose abstinence. *Abstinence* is the commitment not to engage in sexual activity. According to experts, abstinence is the healthiest decision young people can make.

Benefits of Choosing Abstinence

Abstinence is recommended for young people for many reasons. For example, continuous abstinence is the only method that is 100 percent effective for preventing pregnancy, STIs, and HIV/AIDS. Abstinence also allows young people to enjoy dating without the complicated emotions that come with sexual activity.

There are many ways to express affection for another person without sexual activity. Holding hands, hugging, and kissing are ways to show physical affection without sexual activity.

Dating partners can also show affection without physical touch. They can provide each other emotional support and share common interests. They may learn new activities or hobbies together. These are ways to make each partner feel important and respected. Simply telling a partner that you care for them or sharing compliments can show affection.

Influences on Sexual Activity

Many external sources can influence a young person's decision about sexual activity. For example, friends and peers may begin talking about sex. You may hear about older family members engaging in sexual activity. You may see teen sexual relationships portrayed in advertisements, films, and other media. The implied message is that sex is a common part of young people's relationships. This is not true, however. In reality, millions of young people do not have sex.

If they are dating, young people may feel pressured by their dating partners to have sex. Remember that you have the right to say *no* to sexual activity at any time. In a healthy dating relationship, if you say you do not want to engage in sexual activity, your partner should accept your decision and stop pressuring you.

Strategies for Choosing Abstinence

The best way to refuse sexual activity is to set clear boundaries and communicate with your dating partner about your decision to be abstinent. Clearly state that you are not interested in being sexually active. Speak assertively. Sometimes, you may have to leave a situation. You can walk away from people who are pressuring you. This can reduce the other person's ability to continue pressuring you.

To make it easier to use refusal skills, practice ahead of time what you would do and say if pressured to engage in sexual activity. This can make it easier to react in the moment. You can also seek advice from a parent, guardian, or other trusted adult. Finding friends who understand and support your commitment to abstinence can also help you deal with sexual pressure. In addition to refusal skills, various strategies can help you choose abstinence and stick to your decision (**Figure 11.2.5**).

If you are not sure how you feel about sexual relationships, talk to a parent, guardian, adult sibling, or another trusted adult. Trusted adults can help you understand your choices so you can make a thoughtful decision.

Figure 11.2.5 Young people should consider some of the risks that may result from engaging in sexual activity.

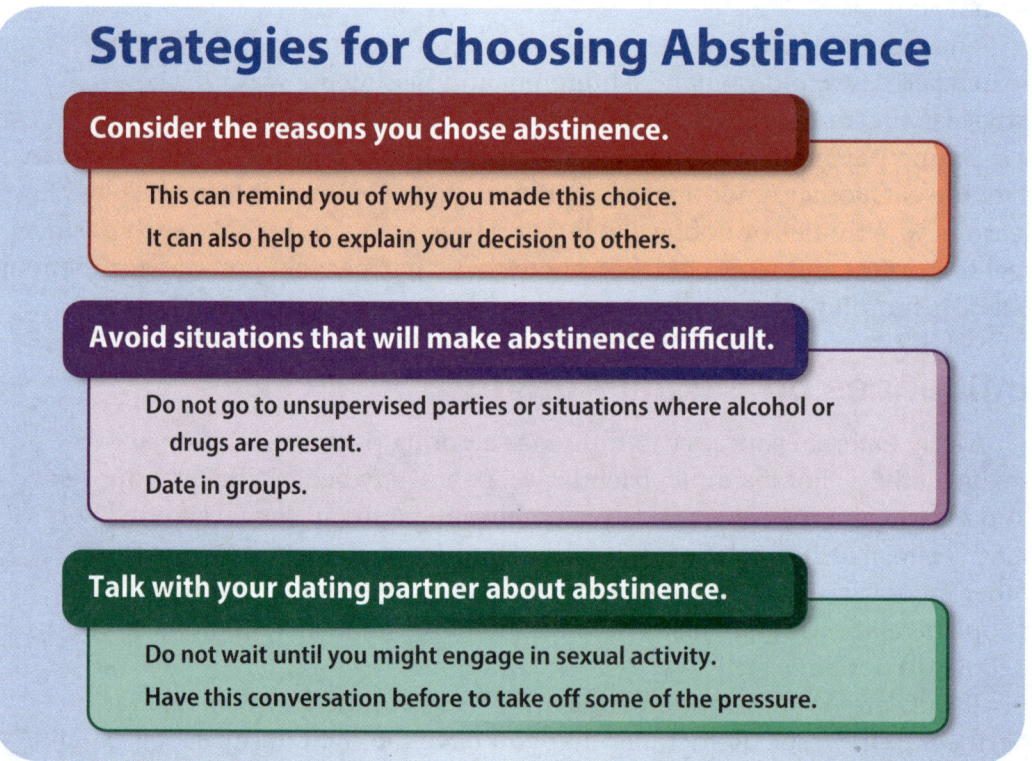

Strategies for Choosing Abstinence

Consider the reasons you chose abstinence.
This can remind you of why you made this choice.
It can also help to explain your decision to others.

Avoid situations that will make abstinence difficult.
Do not go to unsupervised parties or situations where alcohol or drugs are present.
Date in groups.

Talk with your dating partner about abstinence.
Do not wait until you might engage in sexual activity.
Have this conversation before to take off some of the pressure.

Goodheart-Willcox Publisher

CASE STUDY

Cameron and Tyree's Not-So-Magical Relationship

Cameron always imagined that her first real relationship would be magical. Her partner would treat her like a princess and love spending time with her family.

Cameron recently started dating Tyree, and their relationship has been good but not great. Cameron and Tyree go to the movies and play soccer together. Tyree hangs out with Cameron's family, but only for short periods of time. Generally, Cameron enjoys Tyree's company, but she does not feel like a princess.

After three months, the relationship is feeling less and less magical. Cameron feels uncomfortable when Tyree wants her to sit in his lap. Sometimes, Tyree pressures Cameron to send inappropriate text messages. Cameron has let Tyree know this makes her feel uncomfortable, but he has not stopped. Cameron does not know what to do.

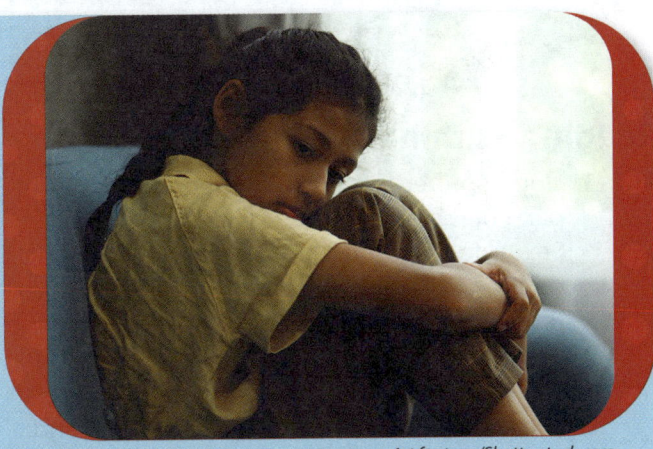

1st footage/Shutterstock.com

 Practice Your Skills — **Set Goals**

Cameron started dating Tyree without any goals related to boundaries, sexual activity, and abstinence. With a partner, discuss SMART goals that Cameron could create that would protect her health now and in the future.

11.2–3 Reading Checkpoint

1. What are the benefits of choosing abstinence?
2. How can young people show affection without sexual activity?
3. Which two strategies do you think are most effective in resisting the pressure to engage in sexual activity?

Lesson 11.2 Review and Assessment

Reading Summary

11.2–1 During puberty, reproductive hormones target parts of the body related to sexual maturity. Sexual feelings and arousal may also develop during puberty.

11.2–2 Physical impacts of sexual activity include pregnancy, STIs, and HIV/AIDS. Emotional and social impacts include feeling overwhelmed, stress about a potential pregnancy or STI, and less focus on individual growth, goals, and other relationships.

11.2–3 Abstinence is the healthiest decision young people can make about sexual activity. It avoids the impacts of sexual activity and promotes heathy relationships. Strategies like refusal skills can help young people remain abstinent.

Critical Thinking

1. **Conclude.** Why might young people find it awkward or difficult to talk or ask questions about their health? How can they make these conversations more comfortable?
2. **Analyze.** What or who influences how young people feel about sexual activity and abstinence?

Develop Your Skills

1. **Advocate for Health.** Create a message in the form of a flyer, poster, social media post, morning announcement message, or other creative product to advocate for abstinence. Include the following in your message: at least five benefits of abstinence, at least five strategies to remain abstinent, at least five ways to show affection that do not involve sexual activity, and other relevant information. With your teacher's permission, display your message.
2. **Make Decisions.** Read the following scenario: *Josh and his dating partner had a conversation early in dating about their decision to be abstinent. Both are focused on their extracurricular activities and future goals, like going to college and traveling around the world. Josh's younger brother is curious about relationships and closely watches them. They both are very respectful of each other's boundaries. Their friends and families support their decision and do not put any pressure on them.* Create a mind map, graphic organizer, or one pager to display how Josh's decision to be abstinent affects himself and others who are close to him.
3. **Communicate with Others.** It is normal to have questions about puberty and sexual activity. Asking questions can help you get accurate information. Create a list of at least five questions you have about puberty and sexual activity. Then, choose a trusted adult with whom you feel comfortable and ask these questions. If you do not feel comfortable initiating this conversation, write a letter to the trusted adult. In your letter, ask your questions and request a time to talk.

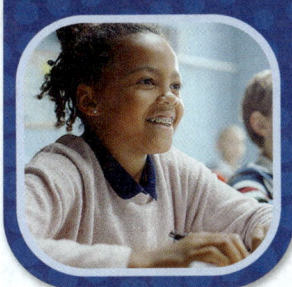

Pregnancy Prevention

Lesson **11.3**

Learning Outcomes

Look for the skills icon ✓ *to practice health skills.*
After studying this lesson, you will be able to
- 11.3–1 **Recognize** pregnancy prevention facts and myths.
- 11.3–2 **Understand** the effectiveness of abstinence in preventing pregnancy.
- 11.3–3 **Identify** barrier methods for preventing pregnancy.
- 11.3–4 **Describe** how hormonal methods and IUDs prevent pregnancy.
- 11.3–5 **Explain** how natural methods and sterilization reduce the risk of pregnancy.

Essential Question

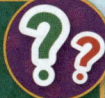

How do various birth control methods reduce the risk of pregnancy?

Reading and Notetaking Activity

Before reading this lesson, draw a rectangle on a separate piece of paper. Write the words *Pregnancy Prevention* in the rectangle. As you read, list general facts about pregnancy prevention above the rectangle. Take notes about different methods of pregnancy prevention below the rectangle.

> Birth control is called contraception
> Reliable information can come from healthcare professionals
>
> **Pregnancy Prevention**
>
> Abstinence—refraining from sexual activity

Goodheart-Willcox Publisher

Key Terms

birth control any method that reduces the risk of pregnancy resulting from sexual intercourse; also called *contraception*

external condom object worn over erect penis during sexual activity

internal condom device similar to a pouch, which is placed inside the vagina

oral contraceptives pills that contain hormones to reduce the chance of pregnancy

birth control patch thin, plastic patch applied to the skin that works like a birth control pill

vaginal ring small, flexible ring that releases hormones to stop ovulation

withdrawal birth control method based on pulling the penis out of the vagina before ejaculation

emergency contraception birth control method used to prevent pregnancy when other birth control has failed

sterilization permanent birth control method in which a medical doctor performs a surgery to prevent sperm and egg from uniting

Lesson image: Gorodenkoff/Shutterstock.com

Introduction

Esmeralda dreams of someday having her own family. She loves her baby brother and likes to babysit him and other children in the neighborhood. Esmeralda looks forward to someday being a parent taking care of her own children. From talking with her parents, however, she knows that pregnancy and parenting are permanent decisions that require much thought and careful planning.

Pregnancy and raising children can be a rewarding and meaningful experience. However, most young people do not yet have the physical and emotional maturity to handle the challenges of pregnancy and parenthood.

Vaginal sexual intercourse always comes with the risk of pregnancy. During vaginal sexual intercourse, a sperm can enter the vagina and reach an egg. The sperm may fertilize an egg, and this can lead to pregnancy.

Sexual activity can lead to sexually transmitted infections (STIs). It also has social and emotional impacts. To guard against these consequences, Esmeralda knows it is important to make responsible sexual decisions.

11.3-1 Myths and Facts About Pregnancy Prevention

In this lesson, you will learn about pregnancy and birth control. **Birth control**, also called *contraception*, is any method that reduces the risk of pregnancy from sexual activity. Many birth control methods exist. They differ in how effective they are. They also differ in whether they protect against STIs.

Many myths exist about pregnancy and sexual intercourse. A good way to avoid falling for myths is to learn the facts about reproduction and pregnancy prevention. Figure 11.3.1 lists some common myths and facts about pregnancy.

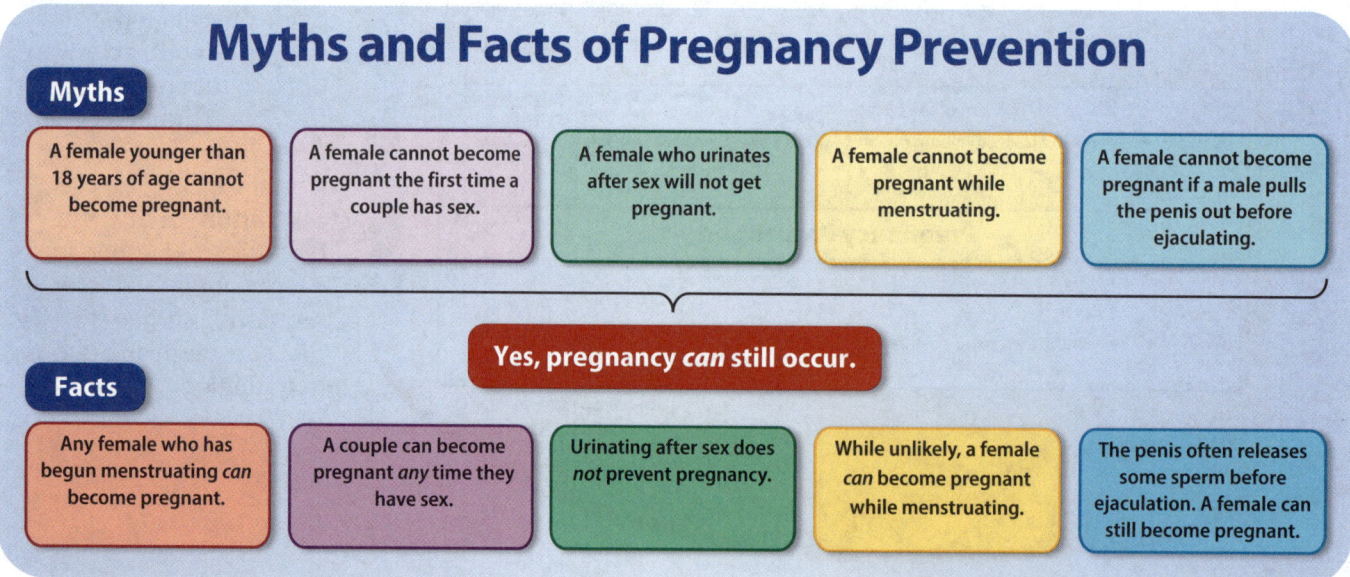

Goodheart-Willcox Publisher

Figure 11.3.1 Widespread myths about pregnancy can cause young people to be misinformed about reproductive health. This can lead to unhealthy behaviors.

The best way to learn the facts about birth control is to talk to a healthcare professional. These trained specialists will be able to discuss birth control methods honestly and objectively. A family doctor or school nurse can also answer these questions.

When using other sources of information, such as a healthcare website, always assess each source's credibility (**Figure 11.3.2**). It is important to have medically accurate information about birth control. A parent, guardian, or other trusted adult can help you find reliable information.

Birth control methods help prevent pregnancy in different ways. Some types of birth control also protect against STIs. Each birth control method has its advantages and disadvantages. When selecting a type of birth control, a person should consider the following:

- personal goals
- the method's effectiveness
- the cost of the method
- whether a doctor's prescription is needed
- whether the method is permanent or reversible
- the method's ease of use
- whether the method helps prevent STIs

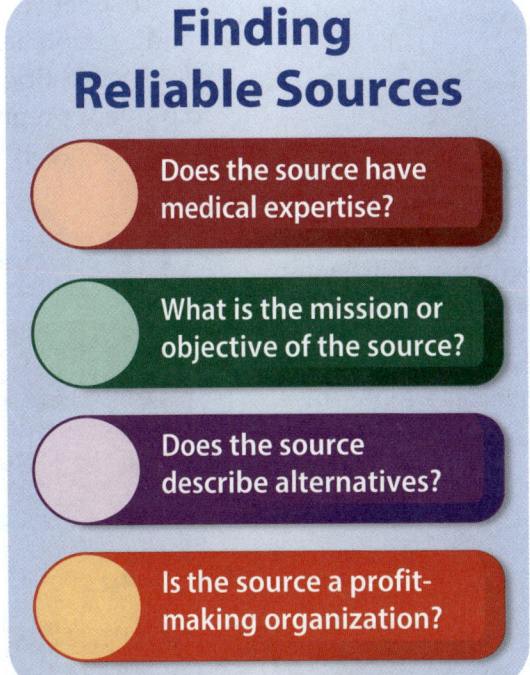

Goodheart-Willcox Publisher

Figure 11.3.2 Illustrated here are some questions you can ask to assess the reliability of a source.

11.3–1 Reading Checkpoint

1. What is one fact about pregnancy you did not previously know? What is one question about pregnancy you still have?
2. List three factors you think are most important to consider when choosing a type of birth control.

11.3–2 Abstinence

The only birth control method that is 100 percent effective in preventing pregnancy is *abstinence*, which is the choice to not engage in sexual activity. Abstinence also prevents STI transmission. It promotes a young person's social and emotional growth.

Abstinence is free and always available. There are no risks involved in using abstinence. It is also a reversible method. This means that people can choose to have children later in life.

Essential Idea

Since it involves not engaging in sexual activity, abstinence is 100 percent effective in preventing pregnancy.

Abstinence has many benefits (Figure 11.3.3). By choosing abstinence, young people learn other ways of showing affection that do not involve sexual activity. Abstinence helps young people focus on their goals. It is guaranteed to prevent pregnancy and STIs. Abstinence is the healthiest, most responsible sexual decision that young people can choose.

Figure 11.3.3
Abstinence is the most responsible sexual decision young people can make. Some of the benefits are listed here.

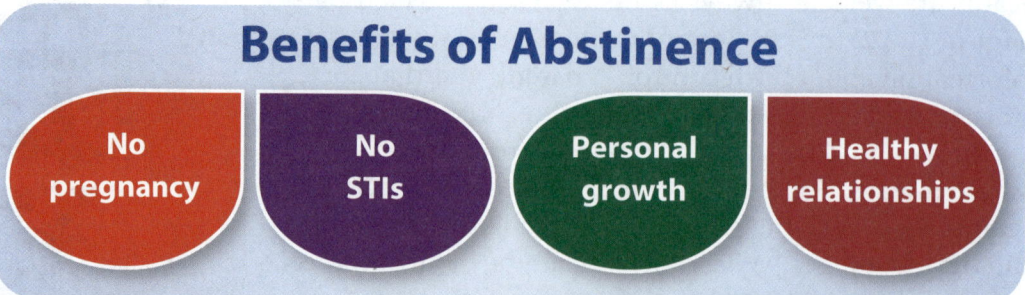

Goodheart-Willcox Publisher

CASE STUDY

Aparna Chooses Abstinence

Aparna and Juan have been dating for a few months. They enjoy spending time together and are having fun getting to know each other. To show their affection, they plan special dates and find opportunities to have fun together. So far, they have not talked about sex. Some of their friends, however, are starting to ask them about it.

A few years ago, Aparna's older sister thought she might be pregnant because her period was late. Aparna and her sister began to discuss the possibility of a child. They thought about the way this would affect her schooling and personal life. Aparna's sister was not pregnant, but it changed the way they both thought about sex.

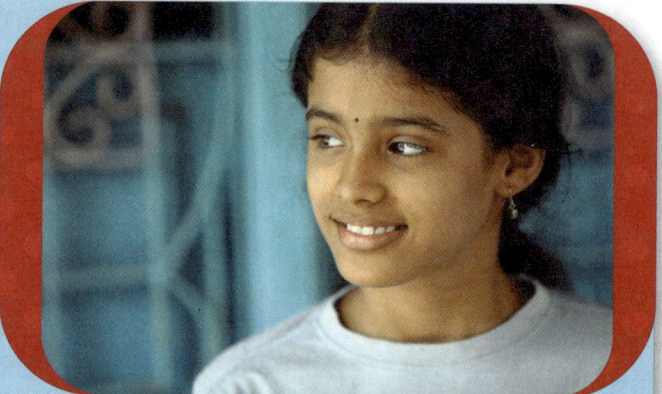

v.s.anandhakrishna/Shutterstock.com

Aparna really likes Juan and wants to continue getting close to him. She also, however, wants to focus on herself, her friends, and her schoolwork. Aparna wants to talk to her parents about her thoughts and feelings. She also wants to set a time to talk with Juan about her boundaries in the relationship.

 Practice Your Skills   **Make Decisions**

With a partner, discuss and record the following:
1. List all the options for Aparna and Juan.
2. List the pros and cons of each option.
3. Based on these pros and cons, make a decision of the best course of action for Aparna and Juan.

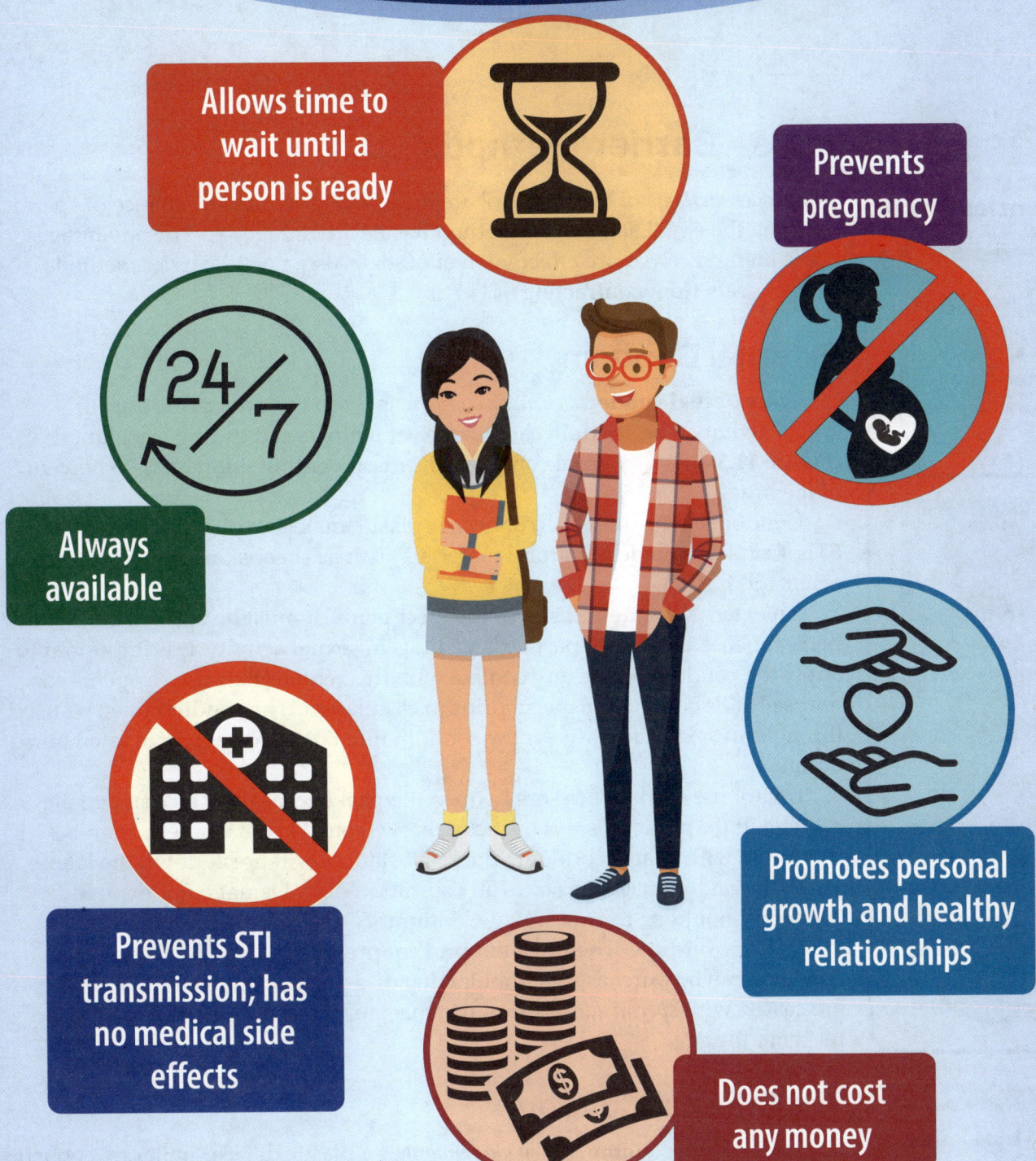

11.3-2 Reading Checkpoint

1. What are the benefits of abstinence?
2. What connection can you make between the information presented and relationships in middle school?

11.3-3 Barrier Methods

Essential Idea

Barrier methods reduce the risk of pregnancy by preventing sperm from reaching an egg.

Barrier methods of birth control are designed to reduce the chance of sperm reaching the egg. Each barrier method has its advantages and disadvantages. Some methods are more effective than others. Also, not all barrier methods protect users from contracting STIs.

External Condom

The **external condom**, or *male condom*, is worn over the penis during sexual activity. The condom catches the semen released during ejaculation (**Figure 11.3.4**). An external condom fails in preventing pregnancy 13 percent of the time.

Condoms made of latex (rubber) or plastic materials also protect against STIs. Condoms made of natural materials such as sheepskin do not protect against STIs.

An external condom fits over the erect penis. It must be applied before the penis touches the sexual partner's genitals in sexual activity. It is important to apply the condom before any contact with the genitals because the penis can release fluids containing sperm prior to ejaculation. The condom must be used throughout sexual activity. A new condom must be used each time intercourse occurs.

Do not use teeth or scissors to open the package, as this can damage the condom. If the package is wet or sticky, throw it out. Do not use petroleum-based lubricants with a latex condom. These substances will break down the latex.

Each condom package states an expiration date. Damaged or expired condoms should be thrown away. Condoms can become dry, brittle, and ineffective over time. They will not prevent pregnancy or STIs. External condoms can be purchased without a doctor's prescription. Some condoms are coated with *spermicide*, a substance that stops sperm from swimming and reaching the egg.

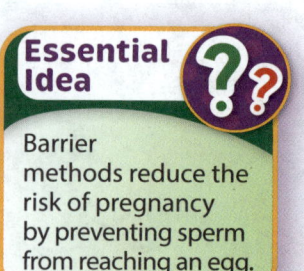
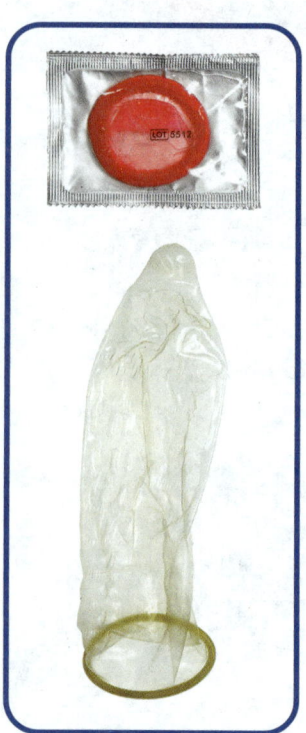

Top to bottom: kaarsten/Shutterstock.com; Dragan Milovanovic/Shutterstock.com

Figure 11.3.4 The external condom is worn over the penis during sexual activity to catch the semen released during ejaculation.

The Internal Condom

The **internal condom**, or *female condom*, is a plastic device similar to a pouch. The internal condom is placed inside the vagina. The internal condom catches semen during ejaculation. An internal condom fails in preventing pregnancy 21 percent of the time. The effectiveness of internal condoms can be improved by using spermicide. Internal condoms also reduce the risk for STIs.

The internal condom must be worn throughout sexual activity. It must be applied before the penis touches a partner's genitals. A new condom must be used each time intercourse occurs. It should not be worn when the partner is also wearing an external condom. The condoms could tear or move out of position, which reduces effectiveness.

Each condom package states an expiration date. Damaged or expired condoms will not prevent pregnancy or STIs. They should be thrown away. Internal condoms can be purchased without a doctor's prescription.

Contraceptive Sponge

The *contraceptive sponge* is made of plastic foam and is about 2 inches in diameter. The sponge is inserted into the vagina and covers the cervix. It helps block sperm from entering the uterus. The sponge contains *spermicide*, which stops sperm from swimming. A contraceptive sponge fails in preventing pregnancy 14–27 percent of the time. It does not protect against STIs. Therefore, a contraceptive sponge should be used in addition to a condom.

Directions on the package describe how to use the sponge correctly. Contraceptive sponges can be purchased without a doctor's prescription.

Diaphragm

The *diaphragm* is a flexible, cup-shaped disk that covers the cervix. The diaphragm helps block sperm from entering the uterus. A diaphragm fails in preventing pregnancy 17 percent of the time. It does not protect against STIs, however. The reusable diaphragm comes with directions for insertion, removal, and care. A person must use it each time intercourse occurs. A diaphragm requires a doctor's exam and prescription.

Cervical Cap

The *cervical cap* is a flexible cup that covers the cervix (**Figure 11.3.5**). Like the diaphragm, the cervical cap helps block sperm from entering the uterus. A cervical cap fails in preventing pregnancy 17 percent of the time. It comes with directions for insertion, removal, and care. The cervical cap requires a prescription from a healthcare professional.

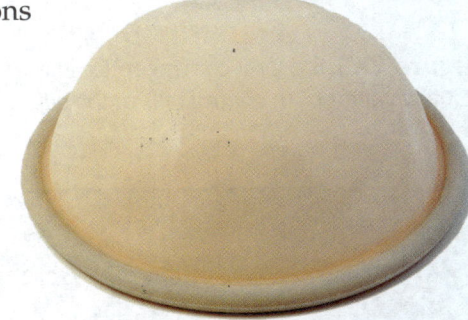

iStock.com/Lalocracio

Figure 11.3.5 The cervical cap is made of silicone and works best for people who have never given birth.

11.3-3 Reading Checkpoint

1. Choose two barrier methods discussed. Explain how they are used, what they protect against, and any other relevant information.
2. Which barrier methods require a prescription from a healthcare professional and which can be purchased at a store?

11.3-4 Hormonal Methods and IUDs

Essential Idea

Hormonal methods and IUDs use the hormones estrogen and progestin to stop ovulation, which helps prevent pregnancy.

Hormones are chemicals in the body that control many body functions, including reproduction. When used medically, the female hormones estrogen and progestin can stop *ovulation*, or the release of an egg. These hormones can also treat some medical conditions, such as severe menstrual pain.

Existing methods use hormones to influence the female reproductive system. However, research is ongoing to identify hormonal methods for male reproductive systems.

Oral Contraceptives

Oral contraceptives, also called *birth control pills* or *the pill*, contain hormones that reduce the risk of pregnancy by preventing ovulation (**Figure 11.3.6**). The pill is taken by mouth, or *orally*, at about the same time every day. The pill fails in preventing pregnancy 7 percent of the time. Skipping even one pill increases the chance of becoming pregnant. Oral contraceptives do not protect against STIs. A prescription from a healthcare professional is needed to purchase the pill.

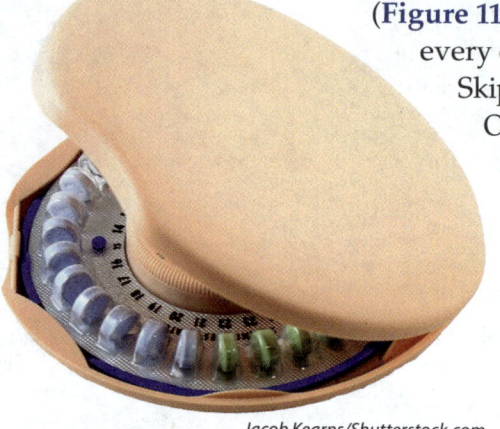

Jacob Kearns/Shutterstock.com

Figure 11.3.6 Oral contraceptives are usually called *birth control pills* or *the pill*.

Birth Control Patch

The birth control patch (often called the *patch*) is a thin, two- to three-inch, plastic patch applied to the skin like a bandage. The patch contains the same hormones as the birth control pill, but hormones in the patch are absorbed through the skin. Each patch comes with directions that should be followed exactly. The patch fails in preventing pregnancy 7 percent of the time.

Vaginal Ring

The vaginal ring is a small, flexible ring inserted into the vagina. The ring contains the same hormones as the birth control pill, but the hormones are absorbed inside the vagina (**Figure 11.3.7**). The vaginal ring comes with directions for storage, insertion, and removal. The vaginal ring fails in preventing pregnancy 7 percent of the time.

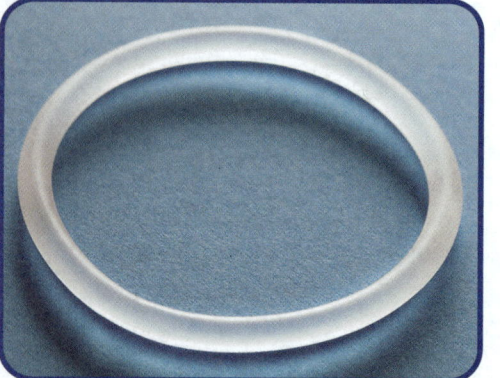

Image Point Fr/Shutterstock.com

Figure 11.3.7 The vaginal ring releases hormones that stop ovulation and thicken cervical mucus.

Birth Control Shot

The *birth control shot* is an injection of a female hormone to stop ovulation. The birth control shot fails in preventing pregnancy 4 percent of the time. A healthcare professional must give the shot every three months.

Birth Control Implant

The *birth control implant* is a flexible, toothpick-sized rod that holds a female hormone that stops ovulation. A doctor inserts the implant under the skin of the upper arm. It can be left in place for three years. The birth control implant fails in preventing pregnancy 0.1 percent of the time.

Intrauterine Device (IUD)

An *intrauterine device (IUD)* is a small, T-shaped device that is inserted into the uterus by a doctor (**Figure 11.3.8**). Two types of IUDs exist: hormonal IUDs and copper IUDs. Hormonal IUDs thicken cervical mucus and prevent ovulation. The copper IUD is thought to interfere with sperm movement, fertilization, and implantation. IUDs last for years. Hormonal IUDs fail in preventing pregnancy 0.1–0.4 percent of the time and copper IUDs fail 0.8 percent of the time. Both types of IUDs can be removed by a doctor if a person wants to become pregnant.

Emergency Contraception

Even when partners agree to use birth control, mistakes can happen. A barrier method might break or move out of place, for example. Sometimes, a person uses a method incorrectly or even forgets to use it.

In these cases, a person might use **emergency contraception** to help prevent pregnancy (**Figure 11.3.9**). This method of birth control can only be used for a few days after sex, however. One form is a copper IUD, which interferes with fertilization and implantation. Another form is a hormone pill. Two common pills are *ella®* and *Plan B One-Step®*. These pills stop ovulation and fertilization.

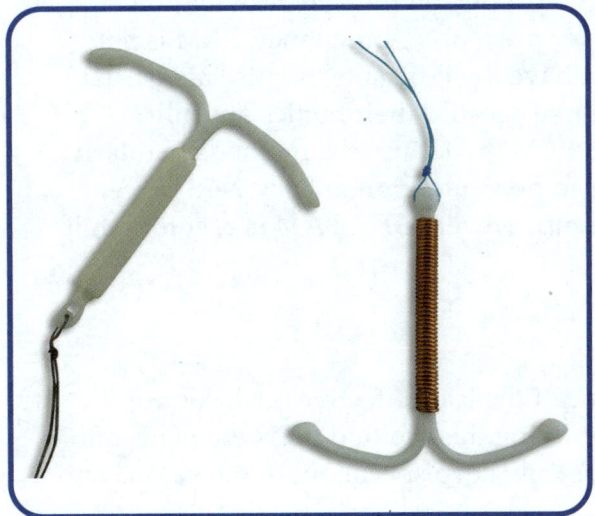

iStock.com/Lalocracio

Figure 11.3.8 IUDs fit inside the uterus. The two types of IUDs are hormonal (on the left) and copper (on the right).

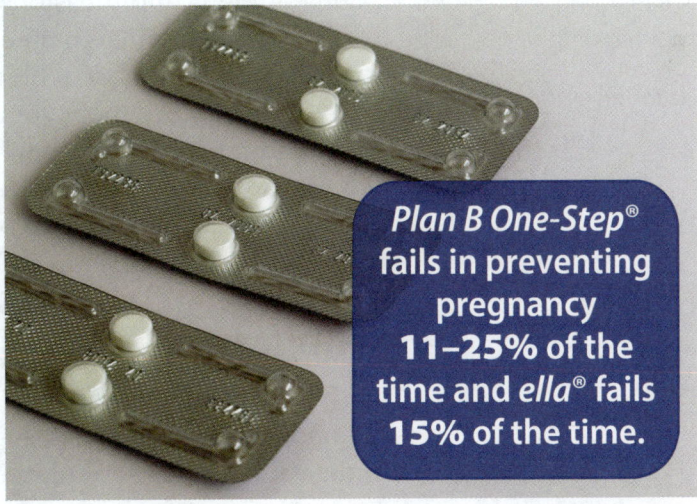

Plan B One-Step® fails in preventing pregnancy 11–25% of the time and *ella®* fails 15% of the time.

Addyvanich/Shutterstock.com

Figure 11.3.9 Emergency contraception can help prevent pregnancy if other forms of pregnancy prevention fail.

How often does *ella®* fail at preventing pregnancy?

Emergency birth control methods do not stop a pregnancy that has already occurred. Emergency birth control also does not reduce the risk of STIs and should not be used regularly. Emergency contraception pills can be purchased without a prescription. A copper IUD needs to be inserted by a doctor.

11.3-4 Reading Checkpoint

1. Choose two hormonal methods discussed. Explain how they are used, what they protect against, and any other relevant information.
2. What method of birth control can be used after sexual intercourse to prevent pregnancy?

11.3-5 Natural Methods and Sterilization

Natural methods of birth control do not use barriers or hormones. Some people prefer these natural methods. Sterilization is a surgical procedure that permanently prevents pregnancy.

Fertility Awareness Method (FAM)

The *fertility awareness method (FAM)* relies on knowing when an egg can be fertilized. Intercourse is avoided in the three to five days before ovulation, and on the first and second day after ovulation. To know when an egg is released, a person can track changes in female body temperature or the mucus in the vagina. A medical professional can help a person track their ovulation.

FAM is only somewhat helpful for preventing pregnancy. FAM is not recommended for those who do not have a predictable, regular menstrual cycle. This includes most young people because their bodies are still developing. Many couples who use FAM do not use the methods regularly and correctly. As a result, FAM fails in preventing pregnancy 2–23 percent of the time. Furthermore, FAM does not prevent STIs. FAM is best for adult couples who are married.

Withdrawal

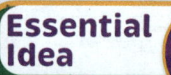

Withdrawal, or *pulling out*, is one of the least effective birth control methods when used alone. A person using this method pulls the penis out of the vagina before ejaculating. This may keep sperm out of the vagina and reduce the risk of pregnancy.

Withdrawal is not an effective method of birth control. Withdrawal is difficult to time. It is not always easy for a person to withdraw during sexual excitement. Fluid containing sperm often leaks from the penis

---

Essential Idea

Natural methods prevent pregnancy by abstaining from sex when an egg can be fertilized or withdrawing the penis before ejaculation. Sterilization permanently prevents pregnancy through surgery.

before ejaculation and can lead to pregnancy (Figure 11.3.10). Withdrawal also does not protect people from STIs.

Sterilization

Sterilization is the only permanent birth control method. It is a surgery performed by a doctor that prevents the sperm and egg from uniting. Sterilization prevents pregnancy, but not STIs.

People who consider this method may not want to have children. Some may already have children but not want to have more children. People may make this choice for genetic, emotional, or financial reasons. People should not choose sterilization if there is any chance they may want children in the future. People should also never feel pressured into sterilization.

Sterilization can be done in both male and female reproductive systems. Male sterilization involves a surgery called a *vasectomy*. In a vasectomy, the *vas deferens* are closed. This prevents sperm from leaving the testes. Vasectomies fail in preventing pregnancy 0.15 percent of the time.

Female sterilization involves *tubal ligation*. In this procedure, the fallopian tubes are cut or sealed. This surgery makes it impossible for sperm to reach an egg. Tubal litigation fails in preventing pregnancy 0.5 percent of the time.

Withdrawal is not an effective pregnancy prevention method.

According to the CDC, withdrawal fails in preventing pregnancy **22%** of the time.

Goodheart-Willcox Publisher

Figure 11.3.10 Rates of pregnancy using withdrawal are high compared to rates using other birth control methods.

How often does withdrawal fail at preventing pregnancy?

11.3-5 Reading Checkpoint

1. Explain the fertility awareness method and why this method is not recommended for young people to prevent pregnancy.
2. Describe sterilization and who it is recommended for.

Lesson 11.3 Review and Assessment

Reading Summary

11.3-1 Birth control are methods for reducing the risk of pregnancy. Healthcare professionals can provide accurate information about birth control.

11.3-2 Abstinence is the most effective method of preventing pregnancy and STIs. Abstinence is the healthiest sexual decision for young people.

11.3-3 Barrier methods prevent sperm from entering the vagina or uterus. These include the external condom, internal condom, contraceptive sponge, diaphragm, and cervical cap.

11.3-4 Hormonal methods use estrogen and progestin to stop the release of an egg. These include oral contraceptives, birth control patch, vaginal ring, birth control shot, birth control implant, intrauterine device (IUD), and emergency contraception.

11.3-5 The fertility awareness method (FAM) prevents pregnancy by scheduling intercourse around ovulation. The withdrawal method involves withdrawing the penis before ejaculation. This method is not effective.

11.3-5 Sterilization is a permanent method of birth control. It involves a procedure called vasectomy for male reproductive systems and tubal ligation for female reproductive systems.

Critical Thinking

1. **Infer.** Why do you think it might be difficult for young people to have conversations with their dating partners about their personal boundaries, sexual activity, and birth control options?
2. **Summarize.** How can young people show affection in a relationship without engaging in sexual activity?
3. **Analyze.** What factors do you think impact a young person's decision to have sex?

Develop Your Skills

1. **Access Information.** Many school and community programs encourage abstinence and help people make responsible sexual decisions. With a partner, research programs that advocate for the reproductive health of young people. Identify one program and research it further. Create a vlog, blog post, flyer, or other product summarizing its mission, service provided, contact information, and other relevant information. Share the program with the class.
2. **Advocate for Health.** With a partner, create a health-enhancing message about pregnancy prevention to other young people creating awareness and a sense of responsibility. In your message, include how choosing abstinence is the most responsible decision for young people. Decide how you will display your message and to whom you want to share it outside of the classroom. Share your message with the class and receive feedback. Make necessary changes, and with your teacher's permission, share your message with the appropriate audience.
3. **Practice Health-Enhancing Behaviors.** In a relationship, practicing abstinence is 100 percent effective in preventing pregnancy and STIs. Abstinence is the healthiest, most responsible choice and it requires a plan. Write down three situations that could influence young people to engage in sexual activity. For each situation, provide alternative activities or behaviors to remain abstinent. Lastly, summarize the importance of assuming responsibility for personal health behaviors.

Glossary/Glosario

English

A

abstinence. Commitment to refrain from sexual activity. (8.4)

abuse. Violent behaviors that cause physical, emotional, sexual, or financial harm to another person. (9.3)

acquired immunodeficiency syndrome (AIDS). Health condition in which the body cannot fight infections. (10.3)

adoption. Action of legally raising another person's biological child. (10.1)

affection. Expression of caring for another person. (9.4)

age of consent. Age at which a person can legally agree to engage in sexual activity. (9.2)

antiretroviral therapy (ART). Treatment for HIV/AIDS in which a combination of drugs is given to control HIV reproduction in the body. (10.3)

arousal. Sexual excitement. (11.2)

B

biological sex. Individual's sex, male or female, as determined by their sex chromosomes. (11.1)

birth control. Any method that reduces the risk of pregnancy resulting from sexual intercourse; also called *contraception*. (11.3)

birth control patch. Thin, plastic patch applied to the skin that works like a birth control pill. (11.3)

breakup. End of a dating relationship. (9.4)

bullying. Repeated aggressive behavior toward someone that causes them injury or discomfort. (9.1)

bystander effect. Situation in which a bystander is less likely to intervene because they think someone else will. (9.1)

bystanders. People who are present at a situation, but do not intervene. (9.1)

Español

abstinencia. Compromiso de abstenerse de la actividad sexual. (8.4)

abuso. Patrón de maltrato físico, emocional, sexual o financiero con violencia hacia otra persona. (9.3)

síndrome de inmunodeficiencia adquirida (SIDA). Afección de salud en la que el cuerpo no puede combatir infecciones y enfermedades. (10.3)

adopción. Acción de criar legalmente al hijo biológico de otra persona. (10.1)

afecto. Expresión de cuidar a otra persona. (9.4)

edad para dar consentimiento. Edad a la que una persona puede aceptar legalmente participar en actividades sexuales. (9.2)

terapia antirretroviral (TARV). Tratamiento para el VIH/SIDA en el que se administra un combinación de drogas para controlar la reproducción del VIH en el cuerpo. (10.3)

excitación. Excitación sexual. (11.2)

sexo biológico. Sexo de una persona, varón o hembra, según lo que determinan los cromosomas sexuales. (11.1)

control de natalidad. Cualquier método que reduce el riesgo de embarazo como resultado de mantener relaciones sexuales; también se conoce como *anticoncepción*. (11.3)

parche anticonceptivo. Parche plástico fino, aplicado a la piel que funciona como una pastilla del control de la natalidad. (11.3)

ruptura. Término de una relación de noviazgo. (9.4)

intimidación. Comportamiento repetido y agresivo hacia alguien que lo causa herida o incomodidad. (9.1)

efecto espectador. Situación en la que un espectador tiene menos probabilidades de intervenir porque cree que alguien más lo hará. (9.1)

espectadores. Personas que están presentes en una situación, pero que no intervienen. (9.1)

The numbers in parentheses following definitions represent the lesson in which the terms appear.

English	Español

C

casual dating. Way of getting to know another person without being in a dating relationship. (9.4)

child abuse. Any intentional act by an adult that causes harm or threatens to cause harm to a child. (9.3)

chlamydia. Bacterial infection known as a "silent" disease because it has few or no symptoms. (10.2)

condom. Device that provides a barrier to pathogens that cause STIs. (10.2)

cyberbullying. Form of bullying using electronic means. (9.1)

D

disability. Condition that reduces a person's ability to do certain tasks. (8.1)

disorder of sex development (DSD). Development process of having an unclear biological sex. (11.1)

E

elder abuse. Behaviors or neglect that cause harm to someone 60 years of age or older. (8.3)

embryo. Mass of cells implanted in the uterus that develops for six weeks following implantation. (8.3)

emergency contraception. Birth control method used to prevent pregnancy when other birth control has failed. (11.3)

emotional abuse. Attitudes or controlling behaviors that harm mental health. (9.3)

erection. State in which the penis lengths and hardens. (11.2)

estrogen. Hormone that triggers growth and development of the female reproductive organs. (8.2)

exclusive. Committed to being romantically involved with only one dating partner. (9.4)

external condom. Object worn over erect penis during sexual activity. (11.3)

F

fertilization. Process by which the sperm and egg combine to create a zygote. (8.3)

C

citas casuales. Manera de conocer otra persona sin ser en una relación de noviazgo. (9.4)

abuso infantil. Cualquier acción intencional de un adulto que causa daño o amenaza causar daño a un niño. (9.3)

clamidia. Infección bacteriana conocido como una enfermedad "silencioso" porque tiene pocos o no síntomas. (10.2)

condón. Dispositivo que proporciona una barrera para patógenos que causan los ITS. (10.2)

ciberacoso. Forma de intimidación que utiliza medios electrónicos. (9.1)

D

discapacidad. Condición que reduce la capacidad de una persona para hacer ciertas tareas. (8.1)

trastorno del desarrollo sexual (DSD). Proceso de desarrollo en la que el sexo biológico no es claro. (11.1)

E

maltrato de ancianos. Maltrato físico, emocional, sexual o financiero o abandono de alguien mayor de 60 años. (8.3)

embrión. Masa de células implantadas en el útero que se desarrolla durante seis semanas después de la implantación. (8.3)

anticoncepción de emergencia. Método anticonceptivo utilizado para prevenir el embarazo cuando otro método anticonceptivo ha fallado. (11.3)

abuso emocional. Actitudes o comportamientos dominantes que dañan la salud mental. (9.3)

erección. Estado en el que el pene se alarga y endurece. (11.2)

estrógeno. Hormona que provoque el crecimiento y desarrollo de los órganos reproductivas femeninas. (8.2)

exclusivo. Comprometido a ser involucrada románticamente con solamente uno pareja de citas. (9.4)

condón externo. Objeto que se usa sobre un pene erecto durante la actividad sexual. (11.3)

F

fertilización. Proceso por el cual el espermatozoide y el óvulo combinan para crear un cigoto. (8.3)

English

fetus. Offspring that develops from the ninth week of pregnancy. (8.3)

financial abuse. Use of money to show power in a relationship and make others act in certain ways. (9.3)

G

gangs. Groups of people who carry out violent and illegal acts. (9.4)

gender. Characteristics a society associates with a particular biological sex. (11.1)

gender identity. Deeply held thoughts and feelings a person has about their gender. (11.1)

gender roles. Behaviors society considers "appropriate" for a certain gender. (11.1)

genital herpes. Viral infection that causes sores on the genitals, mouth, or rectum. (10.2)

gonorrhea. Bacterial infection that mainly affects the genitals, rectum, and throat. (10.2)

group dating. Going out with a group that includes the person one is interested in. (9.4)

growth spurt. Period of rapid physical growth that occurs during puberty. (8.2)

H

harassment. Form of bullying that targets part of someone's identity, such as race, religion, or sex. (9.1)

hate crimes. Threats or violence against someone because of his or her race, ethnic origin, disability, sex, or religion. (9.4)

hazing. Use of pressure to make someone do embarrassing or dangerous activities to be accepted by a group. (9.1)

hepatitis. Potentially severe liver disease caused by different viruses. (10.2)

homicide. Crime of killing another person. (9.4)

homophobia. Hostility, anger, exclusion, and violence directed at LGBTQ+ individuals. (11.1)

hospice care. Type of care given to people who are dying that gives comfort and support to them and their families. (8.1)

human immunodeficiency virus (HIV). Bloodborne virus that infects and kills white blood cells, weakening the body's immune system; can lead to AIDS. (10.3)

Español

feto. Cría que se desarrolla de la novena semana de gestación. (8.3)

abuso financier. Uso del dinero para demostrar poder en una relación y hacer que otras personas actúen de determinada manera. (9.3)

pandillas. Grupos de personas que llevar a cabo acciones violentos e ilegales. (9.4)

género. Características una sociedad asocial con un sexo biológico particular. (11.1)

identidad de género. Pensamientos y sentimientos profundos una persona tiene sobre su género. (11.1)

roles de género. Conductas que la sociedad considera "adecuadas" para cierto género. (11.1)

herpes genital. Infección vírica que produce úlceras en los genitales, la boca o el recto. (10.2)

gonorrea. Infección bacteriana que afecta principalmente los genitales, el recto, y la garganta. (10.2)

citas grupales. Salir con un grupo que incluye la persona uno está interesado. (9.4)

estirón. Período de crecimiento físico rápido que ocurre durante la pubertad. (8.2)

acoso. Forma de intimidación dirigida a una parte de la identidad de alguien, como la raza, la religión o el sexo. (9.1)

crímenes de odio. Amenazas o violencia contra alguien debido a su raza, origen étnico, discapacidad, sexo o religión. (9.4)

novatadas. Uso de presión a hacer que alguien haga activitidades vergonzosas o peligrosas para ser aceptado por un grupo. (9.1)

hepatitis. Inflamación del hígado potencialmente grave causado por diferentes virus. (10.2)

homicidio. Crimen de matar otra persona. (9.4)

homofobia. Hostilidad, ira, exclusión y violencia dirigida a personas LGBTQ+. (11.1)

cuidado de enfermos terminales. Tipo de asistencia dado a las personas que están muriendo que da comodidad y apoyo a ellos y sus familias. (8.1)

virus de inmunodeficiencia humana (VIH). Virus transmitido por la sangre que infecta y mata los glóbulos blancos, debilitando el sistema inmunológico del cuerpo; puede llevar a AIDS. (10.3)

English

human life cycle. Sequence of developmental stages from birth through adulthood. (8.1)

human papillomavirus (HPV). Most commonly contracted STI; causes genital infections and may cause cancer. (10.2)

human trafficking. Form of modern slavery which involves people forcing or pressuring someone to perform a job or service. (9.4)

I

infatuation. Intense romantic feelings for another person that develop suddenly and are usually based on physical attraction. (9.4)

internal condom. Device similar to a pouch, which is placed inside the vagina. (11.3)

intimate partner violence. Abuse that involves two people who are or were in a romantic relationship. (9.3)

L

legal consent. Direct, verbal, freely given agreement that occurs when someone older than the legal age of consent clearly says *yes*. (9.2)

life expectancy. Estimate of how long a person in a particular society is likely to live. (8.1)

life span. Number of years a person lives. (8.1)

long-term non-progressors. People living with HIV whose infection progresses to AIDS very slowly. (10.3)

M

masturbation. Self-stimulation of the sex organ. (11.2)

menstruation. Discharge of some tissue and blood from the uterus. (8.2)

N

neglect. Type of child abuse in which a child's basic physical, emotional, medical, or educational needs are not met by parents or guardians. (9.3)

Español

ciclo de vida humana. Secuencia de las etapas de desarrollo u desde el nacimiento hasta la adultez. (8.1)

virus del papiloma humano (VPH). ITS más comúnmente contratado; causa infecciones genitales y puede causar el cáncer. (10.2)

trata de personas. Forma moderna de esclavitud que implica forzar o presionar a alguien a realizar un trabajo o servicio. (9.4)

enamoramiento. Sentimientos intensos románticos por otra persona que desarrollan bruscamente y son por lo general basado en atracción física. (9.4)

condón interno. Dispositivo similar a una bolsa que se coloca dentro de la vagina. (11.3)

violencia de pareja. Abuso que involucra a dos personas que están o estaban en una relación romántica. (9.3)

consentimiento legal. Acuerdo verbal, directo, y voluntario que ocurre cuando alguien mayor de la edad legal de consentimiento dice que *sí* con claridad. (9.2)

esperanza de vida. Estimación de cuánto tiempo una persona en una sociedad particular es probable a vivir. (8.1)

período de vida. Número de años una persona vive. (8.1)

progresores lentos. Personas que viven con VIH y cuya infección avanza al SIDA muy lentamente. (10.3)

masturbación. Auto-estimulación del órgano del sexo. (11.2)

menstruación. Emisión de algún tejidos y sangre del útero. (8.2)

negligencia. Tipo de abuso infantil en que los necesidades físicos, emocionales, médicos, o educativos básicos de un niño no se cumplen por los padres o guardianes. (9.3)

English

O

obstetrician/gynecologist (OB/GYN). Type of doctor who specializes in pregnancy, labor, and delivery. (8.3)

opportunistic infections. Conditions that occur when pathogens take advantage of a weakened immune system; the cause of death in HIV/AIDS cases. (10.3)

oral contraceptives. Pills that contain hormones to reduce the chance of pregnancy. (11.3)

ovulation. Release of an egg from one of the follicles into the uterus. (8.3)

P

passion. Intense and exciting feeling based on physical attraction. (9.4)

peer abuse. Violent mistreatment of one peer by another. (9.1)

physical abuse. Behaviors that cause physical harm to a person. (9.3)

post-exposure prophylaxis (PEP). Emergency type of ART that a person can take after potential exposure to HIV to reduce risk of transmission. (10.3)

pre-exposure prophylaxis (PrEP). Course of ART that helps prevent HIV transmission; comes in a pill taken daily. (10.3)

prenatal care. Medical care during pregnancy. (10.1)

prenatal development. Changes that occur when a zygote develops during the nine months of pregnancy. (8.3)

primary sexual characteristics. The external and internal reproductive organs. (8.2)

puberty. Stage of life when the body reaches sexual maturity. (8.2)

R

rape. Sexual intercourse that occurs without legal consent. (9.2)

reproductive system. Body system that consists of a group of organs working together to make the creation of new life possible. (8.3)

Español

O

obstetra/ginecólogo (obstetrician/gynecologist, OB/GYN). Tipo de médico que se especializa en el embarazo, el parto, y el alumbramiento. (8.3)

infecciones oportunistas. Afecciones que ocurren cuando los patógenos se aprovechan de un sistema inmunulógico debilitado; causa de muerte en casos de VIH/SIDA. (10.3)

anticonceptivos orales. Pastillas que contienen las hormonas para reducir la probabilidad de embarazo. (11.3)

ovulación. Liberación de un óvulo de uno de los folículos en el útero. (8.3)

P

pasión. Sentimiento intenso y emocionante fuerte basado en atracción física. (9.4)

abuso de pares. Maltrato violento de un par por un otro. (9.1)

abuso físico. Conductas que causan daño físico a una persona. (9.3)

profilaxis posterior a la exposición (PEP). Curso de emergencia de la terapia antirretroviral que puede realizar una persona tras una exposición potencial al VIH para reducir el riesgo de transmisión. (10.3)

profilaxis previa a la exposición (PrEP). Curso de TARV que ayuda a prevenir la transmisión de VIH; viene en una píldora que se toma todos los días. (10.3)

atención prenatal. Cuidado médico durante el embarazo. (10.1)

desarrollo prenatal. Cambios que ocurren cuando se desarrolla un cigoto durante los nueve meses de embarazo. (8.3)

características sexuales primarias. Los órganos reproductivos externos e internos. (8.2)

pubertad. Etapa de la vida cuando el cuerpo alcanza la madurez sexual. (8.2)

R

violación. Relaciones sexuales que ocurren sin consentimiento legal. (9.2)

sistema reproductivo. Sistema corporal que consiste en un grupo de órganos trabajando juntos para hacer posible la creación de una vida nueva. (8.3)

English	Español
S	

safe haven laws. Laws that allow people to leave their babies at certain facilities with no questions asked; also called *safe surrender laws*. (10.1)

school violence. Violent behavior that occurs at any school-related event. (9.4)

secondary sexual characteristics. Features of the mature body other than the reproductive organs. (8.2)

sext. To send sexual content as digital text, a picture, or a video. (8.4)

sexual abuse. Sexual activity to which one person does not or cannot legally consent. (9.3)

sexual activity. Contact that stimulates the external reproductive organs, such as the penis or vagina. (11.2)

sexual assault. Act of threatening, pressuring, or forcing someone into sexual activity. (9.2)

sexual harassment. Verbal or nonverbal sexual attention that occurs without legal consent. (9.2)

sexual orientation. Lasting pattern of romantic and sexual attraction. (11.1)

sexual violence. Sexual behaviors that occur without legal consent. (9.2)

sexuality. A person's biological sex, sexual feelings, sexual orientation, gender identity, and gender expression. (11.1)

sexually transmitted infections (STIs). Infectious diseases spread from one person to another primarily through sexual activity. (10.2)

sibling abuse. Violent behaviors that one sibling inflicts on another sibling. (9.3)

stalking. Following and repeatedly contacting someone in a way that causes the person to feel scared, nervous, or threatened. (9.1)

statutory rape. Crime that takes place when someone over the age of consent engages in sexual intercourse with someone under the age of consent. (9.2)

sterilization. Permanent birth control method in which a medical doctor performs a surgery to prevent sperm and egg from uniting. (11.3)

---

leyes de refugio seguro. Leyes que permite a las personas dejar a sus bebés en ciertas instalaciones sin hacer preguntas; también llamadas *leyes de entrega segura*. (10.1)

violencia escolar. Comportamiento violento que ocurre en eventos relacionados con la escuela. (9.4)

características sexuales secundarias. Características del cuerpo maduro otro que los órganos reproductivos. (8.2)

sext. Enviar contenido sexual en forma de texto digital, una imagen o un video. (8.4)

abuso sexual. Actividad sexual para la cual una persona no da su consentimiento o no puede dar su consentimiento legal. (9.3)

actividad sexual. Contacto que estimula los órganos reproductivos externos, como el pene o la vagina. (11.2)

agresión sexual. Acto de amenazar, presionar u obligar a alguien a tener actividad sexual. (9.2)

acoso sexual. Atención sexual verbal o no verbal que ocurre sin consentimiento legal. (9.2)

orientación sexual. Patrón duradero de atracción romántica y sexual. (11.1)

violencia sexual. Conductas sexuales que ocurren sin consentimiento legal. (9.2)

sexualidad. El sexo biológico, los sentimientos sexuales, la orientación sexual, la identidad de género, y la expresión de género de una persona. (11.1)

infecciones de transmisión sexual (ITS). Enfermedades infecciosas propagada de una persona a otro principalmente a través de la actividad sexual. (10.2)

abuso de hermanos. Comportamientos violentos que un hermano dirige hacia otro hermano. (9.3)

acecho. Seguimiento y contacto reiterado con alguien a través de maneras que provocan que la persona se sienta atemorizada, nerviosa o amenazada. (9.1)

estupro. Crimen que ocurre cuando alguien sobre la edad de consentimiento participa en relaciones sexuales con alguien bajo la edad de consentimiento. (9.2)

esterilización. Método permanente de control de natalidad en el que un médico realiza una cirugía para prevenir que el esperma y el óvulo se unan. (11.3)

English

syphilis. Bacterial infection that develops in stages and causes extremely serious health conditions. (10.2)

T

teen parenthood. Act or process of an teen parents raising a child. (10.1)

teen pregnancy. Pregnancy that occurs during the adolescent years when a person's body is still maturing and growing. (10.1)

terrorism. Use of violence and threats to frighten and control people to promote a political or religious view. (9.4)

testosterone. Hormone that triggers growth and development of the male reproductive organs. (8.2)

transgender. Having a gender identity different from one's biological sex. (11.1)

transphobia. Discrimination and violence directed at people who are transgender. (11.1)

trichomoniasis. Curable infection caused by protozoa. (10.2)

U

upstander. Person who recognizes when a behavior is wrong, takes steps to intervene and stop the behavior, and promotes positive change; also called an *ally*. (9.1)

V

vaginal ring. Small, flexible ring that releases hormones to stop ovulation. (11.3)

W

wet dreams. Ejaculations that occur during sleep starting in male puberty. (11.2)

withdrawal. Birth control method based on the pulling the penis out of the vagina before ejaculation. (11.3)

Z

zygote. Egg that has been fertilized by a sperm. (8.3)

Español

sífilis. Infección bacteriana que se desarrolla en etapas y causa condiciones de salud extremadamente graves. (10.2)

paternidad adolescente. Acto o proceso de un padre adolescente o padres adolescentes criar a un niño. (10.1)

embarazo adolescente. Embarazo que ocurre durante los años de la adolescencia cuando el cuerpo de una persona aún se está madurando y creciendo. (10.1)

terrorismo. Uso de violencia y amenazas para asustar y controlar personas para promover una perspectiva política o religiosa. (9.4)

testosterona. Hormona que provoque el crecimiento y desarrollo de los órganos reproductivos masculinos. (8.2)

transgénero. Tener una identidad de género diferente del sexo biológico de a una persona. (11.1)

transfobia. Discriminación y violencia dirigida a las personas que son transgéneros. (11.1)

tricomoniasis. Infección curable causada por protozoos. (10.2)

espectador activo. Persona que reconoce cuando un comportamiento es incorrecto, toma medidas para intervenir y detener el comportamiento, y promueve un cambio positivo; también denominado un *aliado*. (9.1)

anillo vaginal. Anillo pequeño y flexible que emite hormonas para parar la ovulación. (11.3)

emisión nocturna. Eyaculaciones que ocurren durante el sueño comenzando en la pubertad masculina. (11.2)

retiro. Método de control de la natalidad basado en sacar el pene de la vagina antes de la eyaculación. (11.3)

cigoto. Ovulo que ha sido fecundado por un espermatozoide; también llamada *zigoto*. (8.3)

Index

A

abstinence, 29, 35–37, 90, 135–136, 141–143
    barriers to, 103
    benefits of, 135, 142, 143f
    decision-making process, 94
    influences on sexual activity, 135–136
    reasons for, 36f
    and STIs, 103, 115f, 141
    strategies for choosing, 136
    supporting, 36
abuse, 66, 67
    child. *See* child abuse
    elder, 73–74
    examples of, 67f
    and neglect, 66–77
    preventing, 74–76
    reporting, 75
    responding to, 75
    sibling, 72–73
    signs of, 68f
    stages of, 68
    types of, 67–69
abuse hotlines, 75f
acne, 12, 13, 15
acquaintance rape, 61f
acquired immunodeficiency syndrome (AIDS). *See* HIV/AIDS
adolescence, 3f, 10
adoption, 88, 89
adulthood, 3f
affection, 29, 33–34
agender, 122
age of consent, 55, 56
aggravated sexual assault, 61
AIDS. *See* HIV/AIDS
ally
    bullying and cyberbullying, 51
    LGBTQ+, 128
    sexual harassment, 60
Americans with Disabilities Act (ADA) of 1990, and HIV, 113
antibodies, 110–111
antiretroviral therapy (ART), 109, 114
arousal, 130, 132
ART. *See* antiretroviral therapy
asexual, 125f

B

bacterial STIs, treatment of, 105–106
barrier methods of birth control, 144
bigender, 122
biological sex, 118, 120
birth control, 105, 139, 140–141
    abstinence, 141–143
    barrier methods, 144–145
    cervical cap, 145
    condoms, 144–145
    contraceptive sponge, 145
    diaphragm, 145
    emergency, 147–148
    hormonal methods and IUDs, 146–148
    implant, 147
    intrauterine device (IUD), 147
    natural methods, 148–149
    oral contraceptives, 146
    patch, 146
    shot, 146
    sterilization, 149
    vaginal ring, 146
bisexual, 125f
boundaries
    and abstinence, 136
    in dating relationships, 33–35
    enforcing, 34–35
    respecting others', 63f
breakup, 29, 38
bullying and cyberbullying, 42–54
    consequences, 48–50
    forms of, 45f
    prevention, 52–53
    responding to, 50–51
    signs of, 48f
bystander effect, 42, 51
bystanders, 42, 50

C

cancer, 101, 133
casual dating, 29, 30, 30f
cervical cap, for birth control, 145
child abuse, 66, 70–72
    neglect, 72
    risk factors for, 71f
    sexual, 70f
    signs of, 72f
    types of, 70–71
child neglect, 71
    and abuse, effects of, 71–72
    risk factors for, 71f
    signs of, 72f
Childhelp National Child Abuse Hotline, 75f
childhood, 3f
chlamydia, 97, 99, 105, 105f
chromosomes, 120
cirrhosis, 102, 105f
cisgender, 121
Civil Rights Act of 1991, 128
Civil Service Reform Act of 1978, 128
clitoris, 22f, 23
community violence, 78–86
condom, 97
    external, 144
    internal, 144–145
    and STIs, 104
contraception. *See* birth control
contraceptive sponge, 145
contraceptives, oral, 146
copper IUD, 147
counseling, for sexual assault, 64
cramps, 14
crush, 32
cyberbullying. *See* bullying and cyberbullying
cyberstalking, 47f
cycle of abuse, 68

D

date rape, 61f

Note: Page numbers followed by *f* indicate figures.

dating relationships, 30, 29–39
    boundaries, 33–35
    characteristics of healthy, 30–32
    ending the relationship, 38
    signs of unhealthy, 31*f*
    strategies for healthy, 32–33
dating violence, 69
decision-making process
    for abstinence, 94*f*
    and health issues, 17*f*
    sexual, 94
development, human, 2–8, 4–6
    differences in, 5–6
    factors influencing, 5*f*
    influences on, 5
    prenatal, 20, 25–27
developmental disabilities, 5
diaphragm, for birth control, 143
disability, 2, 5–6
discrimination, 45
    HIV, 113
    LGBTQ+, 126–127
disorder of sex development
    (DSD), 118, 120
domestic violence, 69

E

Education Amendments of 1972, 128
ejaculation, 22
elder abuse, 66, 73–74
embryo, 20, 25
emergency contraception, 139, 147–148
emotional abuse, 66, 67
emotional development, 5, 16–17
emotions, in teen pregnancy, 91
ending a dating relationship, 38
endometrium, 22
environment, human
    development, 5
erection, 22, 130, 132
Erin's Law, 75
estrogen, 9, 12, 22, 131
exclusive, 29, 32
external condom, 104, 139, 144

F

feelings, sexual, 130–138
female condom, 144–145
female puberty, 12, 14–15
female reproductive system, 22–23
fertility awareness method (FAM)
    of birth control, 148
fertilization, 20, 24

fetus, 20, 26
financial abuse, 66, 68
flashing, 67
fluid gender identity, 122
follicle, 22
foster care, 75

G

gang violence, 80–81
gangs, 78, 80
gay, 125*f*
gender, 118, 121
    gender-based violence, 61
    gender binary, 121
    gender expectations, 121
    gender expression, 124
    gender roles, 118, 121
    gender stereotypes, 121
gender identity, 118, 121–122
gender nonconforming, 122
genes, 5
genital herpes, 97, 100–101, 105*f*, 106
genital warts, 133
gonorrhea, 97, 98*f*, 99, 100*f*, 105–106, 105*f*
gossip, 46
grief, 6–7
grooming, in human trafficking, 82
group dating, 29, 32
growth spurt, 9, 10

H

harassment, 42, 45
hate crimes, 78, 83
hazing, 42, 45
health
    and female puberty, 14
    and male puberty, 12
    sexual, 117–150
Health Insurance Portability and
    Accountability Act (HIPAA), 113
healthy dating relationships, 30–32
hepatitis, 97, 101–102
    symptoms of, 105*f*
    treatment of, 107
    vaccine, 104
herpes simplex virus, 100–101
heterosexual, 125*f*
HIPAA, 113
HIV, 110*f*
    antibodies, 110
    medications for risk reduction, 115
    prevention of, 114–115

    testing for, 112–113
    transmission of, 111
HIV/AIDS, 109–116
    and abstinence, 135
    signs and symptoms, 112
    stages of, 112
    treatment for, 114
homicide, 78, 83
homophobia, 118, 126
hormonal IUD, 147
hormones
    and birth control, 146
    in pregnancy, 24
    reproductive, 131
    and sexual activity, 133–134
    and sexual feelings, 132
hospice care, 2, 6
hotlines for abuse, 75*f*
HPV. *See* human papillomavirus
HSV, 100, 101*f*
human development, 2–8
human immunodeficiency virus
    (HIV). *See* HIV/AIDS
human life cycle, 2, 3–4
human papillomavirus (HPV), 97, 101, 104, 105*f*, 106
human trafficking, 78, 81–82

I

implant, for birth control, 147
infancy, 3*f*
infatuation, 29, 32
inhibition, 103
intellectual development, human, 5, 15
intellectual disabilities, 5
internal condom, 104, 139, 144–145
intersex, 120
intimate partner violence, 66, 69–70
intrauterine device (IUD), 147

L

labor trafficking, 81
learning disorders, 5–6
legal consent, 55, 56–58
lesbian, 125*f*
LGBTQ+, 125
    discrimination and violence
        against, 126–127
    federal laws protecting, 128
    questions about sexuality, 126
    social support for, 127
    support for young people, 128
life cycle. *See* human life cycle
life expectancy, 2, 4

life span, 2, 4
long-term non-progressors, in HIV, 109, 112
love, 32

M

male condom, 144
male primary sexual characteristics, 10
male puberty, 12
male reproductive system, 21–22
mandated reporters of abuse, 75
masturbation, 130, 132
Matthew Shepard and James Byrd, Jr. Hate Crimes Prevention Act, 128
Medicaid, 93
medicine, for HIV risk reduction, 115
menarche, 14
menstrual cups, 14
menstrual cycle, 23
menstruation, 9, 14, 23, 132
mental abuse, 67
middle childhood, 3f, 10
mood disorders after pregnancy, 27

N

National Domestic Violence Hotline, 75f
National Human Trafficking Hotline, 82f
National Sexual Assault Hotline, 64
National Teen Dating Abuse Hotline, 75f
needle sharing, and STIs, 111, 113, 114, 115
neglect, 66, 71–72
nonbinary, 122
nonverbal sexual harassment, 59

O

obstetrician/gynecologist (OB/GYN), 20, 24
opportunistic infections, 109, 112
oral contraceptives, 139, 146
ovaries, 22
ovulation, 20, 23, 146

P

papillomavirus, human (HPV), 101
parenthood, teen. *See* teen parenthood
passion, 29, 32
patch, for birth control, 146
peer abuse, 42, 43
peer pressure, 17–18, 34
peers, and puberty, 16
penis, 21, 22
physical abuse, 66, 67
physical disabilities, 5
placenta, 26
platonic relationship, 31
post-exposure prophylaxis (PEP), 109, 115
postpartum changes, 27
postpartum depression, 27
power and control wheel of abuse, 68f
pre-exposure prophylaxis (PrEP), 109, 115
pregnancy, 24, 133, 134f
    and abstinence, 135
    changes during, 26
    healthy behaviors, 92f
    options for, 89
    preventing, 35, 139–150
    teen. *See* teen pregnancy
prenatal care, 88, 91
prenatal development, 20, 25–27
preventing pregnancy, 139–150
primary sexual characteristics, 9, 10, 131–132
progesterone, 22
promoting health to prevent abuse, 74
pronouns and gender identity, 122
prostate, 21f, 22
psychological abuse, 67
puberty, 3f, 9, 10, 129
    changes during, 9–19
    differences in development, 11–12
    emotional development, 16–17
    female, 12, 14–15
    intellectual development, 15
    male, 12
    physical development, 10–15
    sexual changes, 131–132
    social development, 16–17
pulling out, method of birth control, 148–149

R

rape, 55, 61
refusal skills
    and abstinence, 136
    sexual activity, 103f
    sexual pressure, 37–38

Rehabilitation Act of 1973, 113
relationships
    boundaries, 33–35
        dating, 29–40, 32–33, 38
        and sexual activity, 133–134
reproduction, human, 20–28
reproductive health, 117–150
reproductive hormones, 10, 131
reproductive system, 20, 21–23
risk factors
    for teen pregnancy, 90
    for violent behavior, 43f
romantic relationships. *See* dating relationships
rumors, 46

S

safe haven laws, 88, 89
safe surrender laws, 89
same-sex marriage, 128
sanitary pads, 14–15
school violence, 78, 79–80
secondary sexual characteristics, 9, 10, 132
semen, 22
sex trafficking, 81
sexting, 29, 34, 133–134
sexual abstinence. *See* abstinence
sexual abuse, 66, 67
sexual activity, 130, 133–134
    abstaining from, 35–37, 135–136
    impacts on health, 133–134
    and STIs, 98
    unwanted, 55–65
sexual assault, 55, 56, 61–64
    examples of, 61f
    impact of alcohol or other substances, 56f
    impacts on health, 62f
    preventing, 63
    responding to, 64
    supporting survivors, 64
sexual characteristics, 9, 10, 131–132
sexual harassment, 55, 56, 58–59
    effects of, 59f
    preventing and responding to, 59–60
    stopping, 60f
sexual intercourse, 24
sexual orientation, 118, 125
sexual reproduction, human, 24
sexual violence, 55, 56–58, 61
sexuality, 118–129

sexually transmitted infections (STIs), 97–108
   and abstinence, 135
   bacterial, 105–106
   causes, 98
   preventing, 35, 103–104
   resources, 107
   symptoms of, 105*f*
   treatment of, 105–107
   viral, 106–107
shot, for birth control, 146
social development, 5, 16–17
Special Supplemental Nutrition Program for Women, Infants, and Children (WIC), 93
sperm, 21
spermicide, 144, 145
sponge, contraceptive, 145
spousal violence, 69
stages of abuse, 68
stalking, 42, 45
statutory rape, 55, 62
sterilization, for birth control, 139, 149
STIs. *See* sexually transmitted infections
straight, sexual orientation, 125*f*
survivors of sexual assault, 64
syphilis, 97, 100, 105, 105*f*

T

tampons, 14–15
tattoos, 111, 114
teen parenthood, 88–96
teen parents, resources for, 93
teen pregnancy, 88–96
   challenges of, 91–92
   impacts of, 91*f*
   options for, 89
   risk and protective factors, 90
terrorism, 78, 83–84
testosterone, 9, 12, 21, 131
Title IX of Education Amendments of 1972, 128
toddler years, 3*f*
trafficking, human, 78, 81–82
transgender, 118, 122
transmission of HIV, 111
transphobia, 118, 126
trichomoniasis, 97, 99, 105, 105*f*
tubal ligation, for birth control, 149

U

umbilical cord, 26
upstander, 42, 51, 60
urethra, 21*f*, 22
uterus, 22

V

vaccine, 104
vagina, 22
vaginal ring, 139, 146
vas deferens, 21, 22, 149
vasectomy, 149
verbal abuse, 67
verbal sexual harassment, 58
violence, 41–86
   community, 78–86
   gang, 80–81
   intimate partner, 69–70
   LGBTQ+, 126–127
   prevention strategies, 79–80
   responding to and preventing, 85
   school, 78, 79–80
violent behavior, 43, 43–44*f*
violent extremism, 83–84

W

wet dreams, 130, 132
WIC, 93
withdrawal method of birth control, 148–149

Z

zygote, 20, 24, 25